Firuz Shukurov
Fariza Halimova

PHYSIOLOGY IN DIAGRAMS AND DRAWINGS

Firuz Shukurov
Fariza Halimova

PHYSIOLOGY IN DIAGRAMS AND DRAWINGS

ScienciaScripts

Imprint

Any brand names and product names mentioned in this book are subject to trademark, brand or patent protection and are trademarks or registered trademarks of their respective holders. The use of brand names, product names, common names, trade names, product descriptions etc. even without a particular marking in this work is in no way to be construed to mean that such names may be regarded as unrestricted in respect of trademark and brand protection legislation and could thus be used by anyone.

Cover image: www.ingimage.com

This book is a translation from the original published under ISBN 978-620-5-51354-5.

Publisher:
Sciencia Scripts
is a trademark of
Dodo Books Indian Ocean Ltd. and OmniScriptum S.R.L publishing group

120 High Road, East Finchley, London, N2 9ED, United Kingdom
Str. Armeneasca 28/1, office 1, Chisinau MD-2012, Republic of Moldova, Europe
Printed at: see last page
ISBN: 978-620-7-62343-3

F.A. SHUKUROV, F.T. HALIMOVA.

PHYSIOLOGY DIAGRAMMATICALLY

Shukurov F.A., Halimova F.T.
Physiology in diagrams and drawings: textbook

The textbook presents sections on the physiology of the cardiovascular system, blood and respiration in accordance with the programme. The textbook consists of three sections. The first section contains schemes that reveal electrical phenomena in the heart, physiological properties of the heart muscle, heart automatism, hemodynamic function of the heart, structure of the cardiac cycle, regulation of the heart, basic laws of hemodynamics, blood pressure and regulation of blood circulation. The second section contains schemes revealing the issues of blood physiology: blood properties; blood form elements, haemoglobin, its types and compounds; coagulation and blood groups. The third section contains schemes revealing questions of physiology of respiratory system: external respiration; indices of pulmonary ventilation; intrapleural pressure; blood gases; gas exchange in lungs and tissues; processes occurring in capillaries of small and large circle of circulation and regulation of respiration.

The manual is designed for students of medical and biological faculties and medical universities.

PREFACE

This textbook has been prepared for publication by the Head of the Department of Normal Physiology of the Tajik State Medical University named after Abuali ibni Sino, Academician of the Russian Ecological Academy, Doctor of Medical Sciences, Professor F.A. Shukurov and Doctor of Medical Sciences, Associate Professor F.T. Halimova. Explanations for each scheme are presented in an accessible language, which ensures the assimilation of material on the relevant issues of physiology. 50 years of pedagogical experience of Shukurov F.A. and 20 years of experience of Halimova F.T. allowed to present the materials of all sections systematically and in an accessible language, which contributes to better assimilation. The use of this textbook allows to study more deeply the mechanisms underlying the functions of all systems. The use of schemes of this manual and explanations to them will allow students to understand the issues of all levels set out in the "Notebook for laboratory classes and independent work on normal physiology"

IRRITANTS. LAWS OF IRRITATION OF EXCITABLE TISSUES

Classification of stimuli by strength

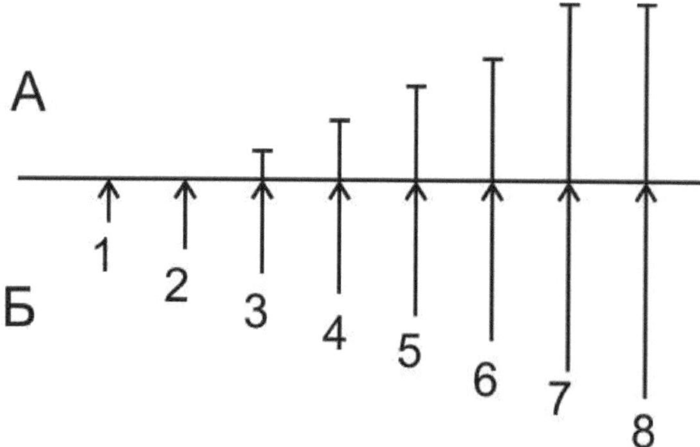

Classification of stimuli by strength: A - magnitude of response, B - stimulus strength: 1,2 - subthreshold stimuli, **3 - threshold stimulus,** 4-6 - supra-threshold, (submaximal) stimuli, **7 - maximal stimulus**, 8 - supramaximal stimuli. It should be noted that one threshold stimulus and one maximum stimulus are noted for each tissue. The threshold stimulus is the smallest stimulus that causes a tissue response for an infinite time of its action. The maximum stimulus is the smallest stimulus force that causes the maximum tissue response. At action of supramaximal stimuli there can be a maximum tissue response, there can be a decrease in the response until it disappears completely.

Force-time curve

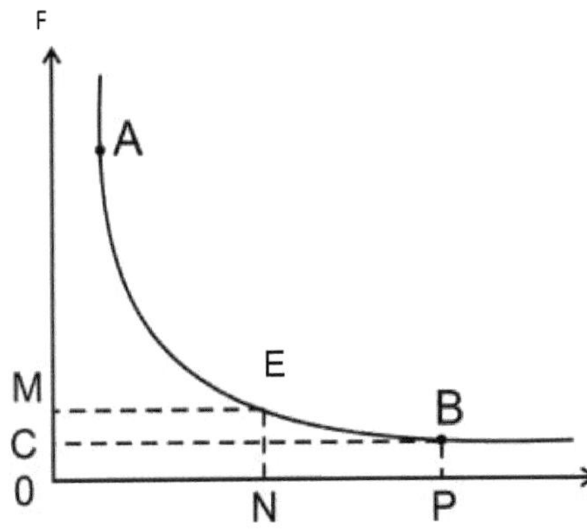

A force-time curve reflecting the dependence of the stimulus strength (F) on the time of its action (t). This dependence is inversely proportional within A-B: the greater the stimulus strength, the shorter its action time. The following indices can be determined from this curve: threshold force or rheobase (OS), useful time (RT) and chronaxy (ON). Useful time is the minimum time that a threshold force must be applied to elicit a tissue response. Chronaxia is the minimum time that two rheobases must be acted upon to produce a tissue response (chronaxia is the useful time when two rheobases are acted upon). Algorithm for determining chronaxia: 1)find a point on the force-time curve where the curve is parallel to the force-time axis (point B), 2) draw from this point a parallel line to the time axis until it intersects with the force axis (point C) and find the rheobase (OS), 3) double the rheobase (OM), 4) from point M draw a parallel line to the time axis until it intersects with the force-time curve (point E), 5) lower the perpendicular from point E to the time axis (point N). The segment ON corresponds to chronaxy. Threshold force (rheobase) and chronaxia are a measure of excitability: the greater the rheobase and chronaxia, the less excitability of the tissue.

The law of the rate of increase of stimulus strength

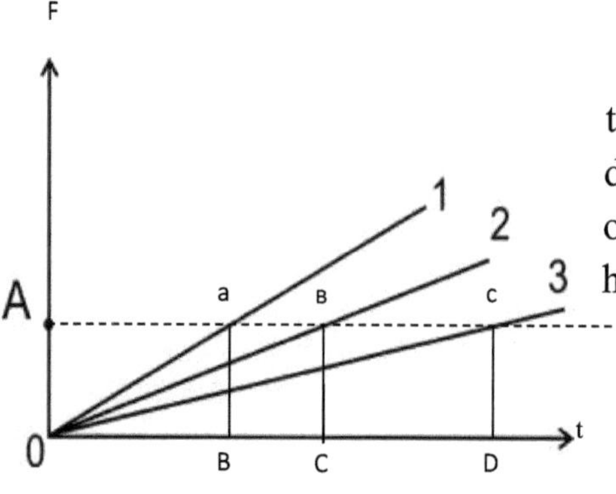

This diagram shows three tissues with different threshold rate of stimulus intensity: the highest threshold rate of stimulus intensity for the first tissue and the lowest for the third tissue. One of the laws of irritation of excitable tissues is the law reflecting the dependence of tissue excitability on the rate of increase of the stimulus force: the lower the threshold rate of increase of the stimulus force, the greater the tissue excitability. On the diagram the third tissue has the highest excitability. To determine the rate of increase of the stimulus strength, we need to take any stimulus strength (OA). From point A we draw a straight line parallel to the time axis to the intersection of 1 (a), 2 (c) and 3 (c). From each point, draw a perpendicular to the time axis. The rate of increase of the stimulus force for the first tissue will be the ratio OA/OV, for the second tissue the ratio OA/OC and for the third tissue the ratio OA/OD. The numerator is the same in all ratios and the denominator is largest for the third ratio, so the smallest rate of increase in stimulus strength is for the third tissue and the largest is for the first tissue.

Dependence of excitability on chronoxia and rate of increase in stimulus strength

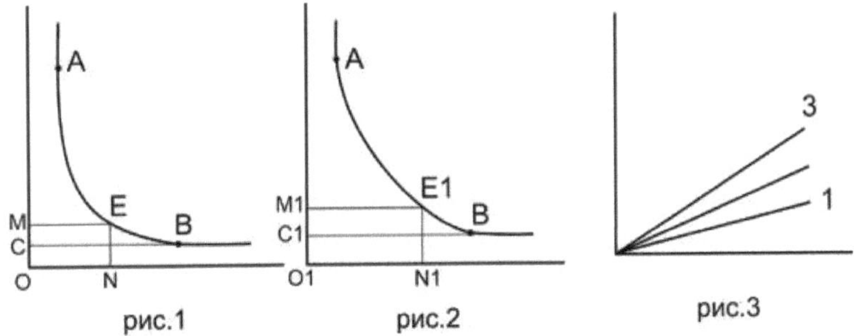

Figure 3 shows the threshold rate of stimulus intensity for the three tissues: the highest rate of stimulus intensity for the third tissue (this tissue has the lowest excitability) and the lowest rate of stimulus intensity for the first tissue (this tissue has the highest excitability). Figures 1 and 2 show force-time curves, one of which reflects the excitability of the third tissue and the other the first tissue (Figure 3). To determine whether the force-time curve corresponds to the first or third tissue, it is necessary to determine the rheobase (threshold force) and chronaxia on each force-time curve. Using the algorithm for determining chronaxia, we find in Figures 1 and 2: 1) find point B; 2) find the rheobase (OS and O1C1); 3) double the rheobase (OM and O1M1); 4) find point E and E1; and 5) find the chronaxia (ON and O1N1). Thus, the greatest chronaxia and rheobase in Fig. 2, i.e., the force-time curve in this figure reflects the excitability of the third tissue in Fig. 3: the greater the chronaxia and rheobase, the greater the rate of increase of the stimulus force.

BIOPOTENTIALS

Different membrane states

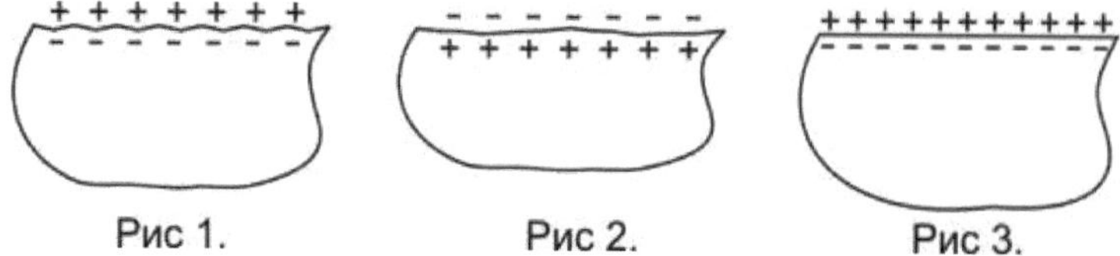

Рис 1.   Рис 2.   Рис 3.

These figures show membranes corresponding to three functional states of the tissue: rest (Fig.1), excitation (Fig.2) and inhibition (Fig.3). Fig.1 shows the state of membrane polarisation, when positive charges accumulate on the outer surface and negative charges on the inner surface. This charge distribution is observed in the resting state. In this case, the resting membrane potential (RMP) is registered, the value of which varies in the range of -70-90 mv. The sign "-" in front of the MPP value indicates that negative charges accumulate on the inner surface of the membrane in the resting state. Fig. 2 shows the state of membrane depolarisation, when negative charges accumulate on the outer surface and positive charges accumulate on the inner surface. This distribution of charges is observed in the state of excitation. In this case, the membrane action potential (MAP) is registered, the value of which varies within +100 +120 mv. The sign "+" in front of the MPP value indicates that in the state of excitation positive charges accumulate on the inner surface of the membrane. Fig.3 shows the state of membrane hyperpolarisation, when positive charges accumulate on the outer surface (more than in the resting state) and negative charges accumulate on the inner surface. Such distribution of charges is observed in the state of inhibition.

Phases of the membrane action potential (MAP)

This figure shows the phases of the membrane action potential (MAP). 80 mV is the value of the resting membrane potential (RMP). When a stimulus is applied to a tissue, an MPP occurs: the MPP decreases to 0 (there are no charges on the membrane surface) and then the membrane is recharged (negative charges accumulate on the outer surface and positive charges on the inner surface) to +30 mv. Thus the value of MPD corresponds to +110 mv (-80 and +30). The following phases are distinguished in the MPD: 1 - depolarisation threshold (A) - occurs as a result of slow entry of sodium ions into the cell - in this case MPP decreases to the critical

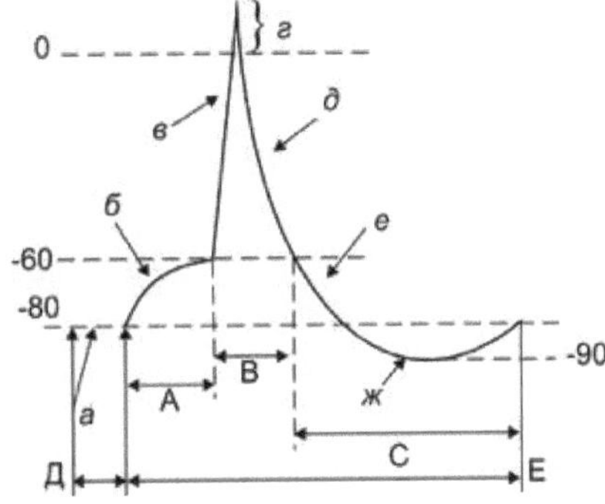

level of depolarisation (CUD -60 mv - this is the value of MPP, at which there is no repulsive force of positive charges on the membrane surface) and the volley entry of sodium ions into the cell begins. The difference between MPP and CUD (in this case 80-60=20) affects the magnitude of the threshold force (tissue excitability): the greater this difference, the greater the threshold force and the less excitability of the tissue; 2 - peak MPP (B), which consists of two periods - depolarisation period (c - arises due to rapid entry of sodium ions) and repolarisation period (e - arises due to the operation of the sodium pump, due to which sodium ions leave the cell against the gradient); 3 - trace potential phase (C), which consists of two periods: period of trace depolarisation (f - from KUD to MPP) and period of trace hyperpolarisation (g - increase in MPP to -90mv due to increased permeability of potassium ions and greater potassium release from the cell compared to what it was before the stimulus action)

Changes in excitability during different phases of MAP

This figure shows the change in tissue excitability at the onset of MPD. The normal phase of excitability corresponds to the resting state (MPP - - 80mv) and is taken as 100%. The phase of depolarisation threshold

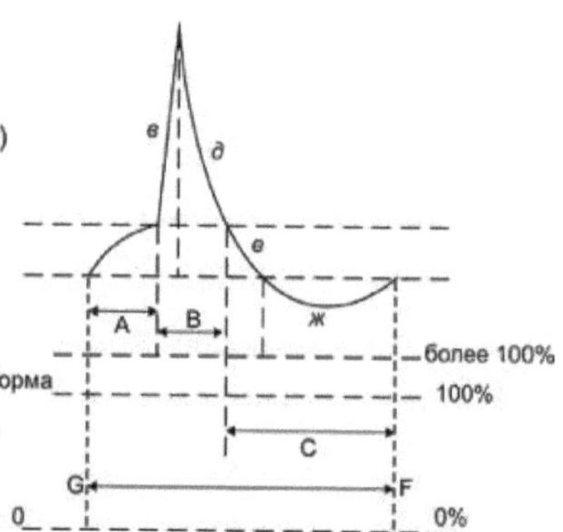

(A) and trace depolarisation (Ce) corresponds to increased excitability (more than 100%) - this supernormal phase of excitability, or exaltation. The period of MPD peak depolarisation (Vv) corresponds to zero excitability (0%) - this absolute refractory phase of excitability - complete absence of excitability. The period of MFD peak repolarisation (Vd) and trace hyperpolarisation (Cj) corresponds to a decrease in excitability (less than 100% but more than 0%) - this is a relative refractory phase of excitability. Thus, during MFD (G-F), tissue excitability can be increased (during the phase of depolarisation threshold and trace depolarisation), decreased (during the repolarisation phase of MFD peak and trace hyperpolarisation), and completely absent (during the depolarisation phase of MFD peak).

Characterisation of excitability at different points in the MAP phase

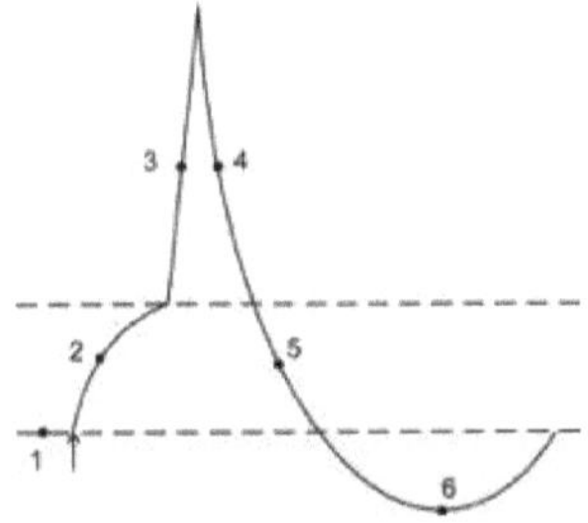

This diagram shows changes in tissue excitability at rest (1) and at different points of the membrane action potential (MAP - 2-6). At point 1, the tissue is at rest - normal tissue excitability is observed. At point 2 (depolarisation threshold phase) and 5 (trace depolarisation) the tissue excitability is increased (supernormal excitability phase, or exaltation) - in this case the tissue can react to subthreshold stimuli. At point 3 (period of depolarisation of the MAP peak), tissue excitability is completely absent (absolute refractory phase of excitability) - in this case, the tissue does not react to stimuli at all. At point 4 (period of repolarisation of the MFD peak) and 6 (trace hyperpolarisation), excitability is below normal (relative refractory phase of excitability) - in this case the tissue reacts to submaximal (supra-threshold), maximal and supra-maximal stimuli and does not react to threshold and sub-threshold stimuli.

MUSCLE PROPERTIES

Motor unit

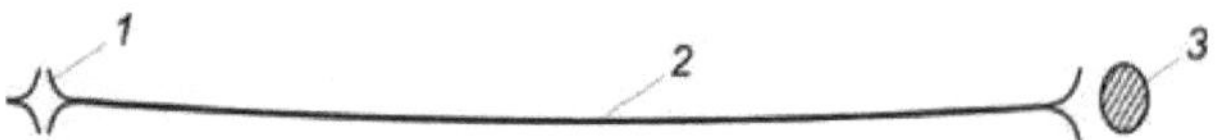

This scheme reflects the motor unit, which consists of the following elements: 1 - motoneuron localised in the anterior horns of the spinal cord; 2 - efferent nerve; 3 - skeletal muscle.

Transverse section of myofilaments

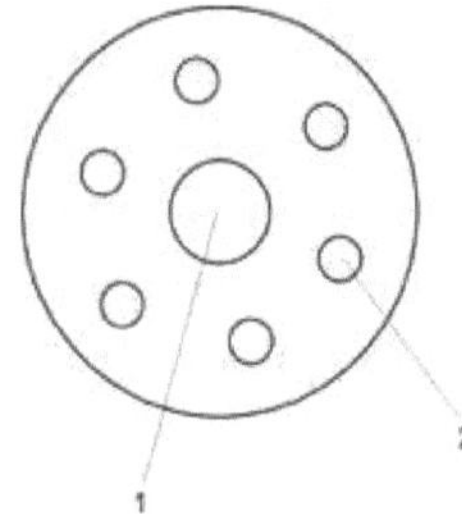

The diagram shows a cross section of a single myofilament, which consists of one thick myosin fibre(1) and six thin actin fibres (2)

Types and types of muscle contraction

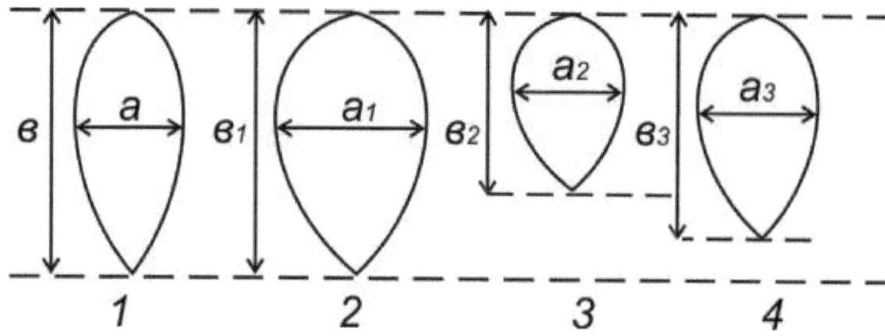

This diagram shows the types of skeletal muscle contraction: 1 - muscle at rest; 2 - isometric muscle contraction. In this type of contraction there is an increase in tension (the cross-section of the muscle a1 increases more than a), the length of the muscle does not change (c=v1); 3 - isotonic contraction. In this type of contraction there is a shortening of the muscle fibre length (c2 is less than c), the cross-section does not change (a=a2); 4 - auxotonic contraction, or mixed type. In this case, there is a shortening of the muscle fibre (c3 is less than c) and an increase in the cross-section (tone): a3 is greater than a.

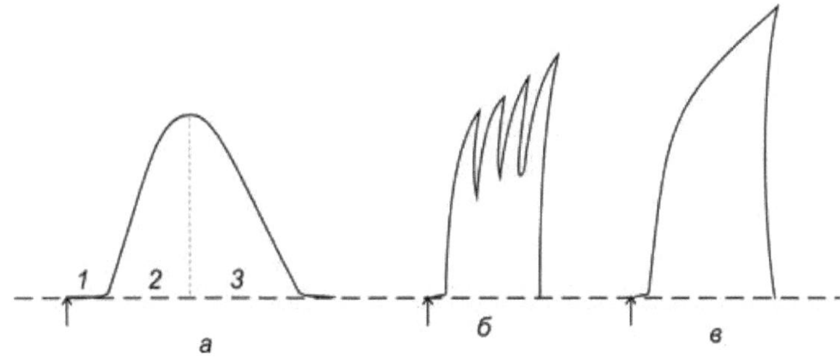

The diagram shows the types of muscle contraction: single muscle contraction (a) and tetanic contraction (b - serrated tetanus, c - smooth tetanus). A single contraction occurs in response to a single stimulus. In this case, three phases are distinguished: 1 - latent, or hidden phase - from the moment of irritation to the beginning of contraction; 2 - contraction phase; 3 - relaxation phase. In the latent phase the following processes take place: membrane depolarisation-appearance of MMPs-propagation of the MMP peak to T-systems-exit of calcium ions from cisternae and its connection with troponin-change in the conformation of troponin-retreat of tropomyosin into the groove of actin filaments-connection of the head of the cross-bridge with actin with the formation of the actomyosin complex-decomposition of ATP. In the phase of muscle contraction due to ATP energy, periodic rupture of the cross-bridge occurs, which leads to sliding of actin filaments along myosin (muscle contraction). In the relaxation phase, the following processes occur: less ATP energy-work of the calcium pump-entry of calcium ions into the cisternae-return of troponin to its original conformation-exit of tropomyosin from the groove of actin filaments-disengagement of the cross-bridge head from actin-return of actin filaments to their original position (relaxation). A thetanic contraction is a strong and prolonged muscle contraction resulting from the action of a rhythmic stimulus. Depending on the frequency of the rhythmic stimulus, a distinction is made between serrated (5-10 Hz) and smooth (more than 15 Hz or more) tetanus.

Skeletal muscle and myocardial excitability

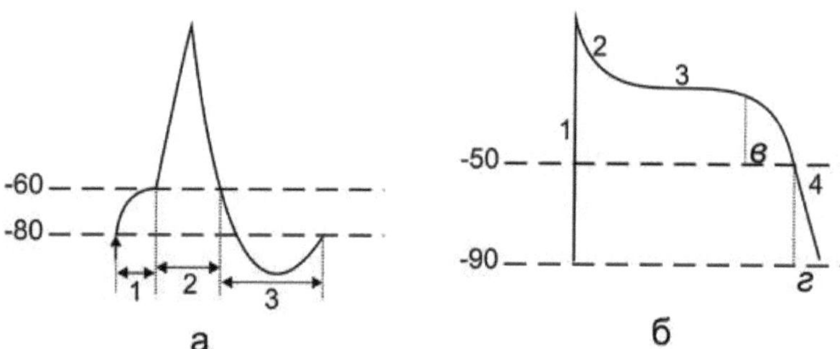

The diagram shows the MEPs of skeletal muscle (a) and myocardium (b). Skeletal muscle MEPs show the following phases: depolarisation threshold (1), MEP peak (2) and trace potential (3). Cardiomyocyte MEPs show the following phases: depolarisation phase (1), early or fast repolarisation (2), plateau (3) and late or slow repolarisation (4): *4c* corresponds to the relative refractory phase of excitability; *4g* corresponds to the super normal phase of excitability.

Structure of myofilaments and T-systems

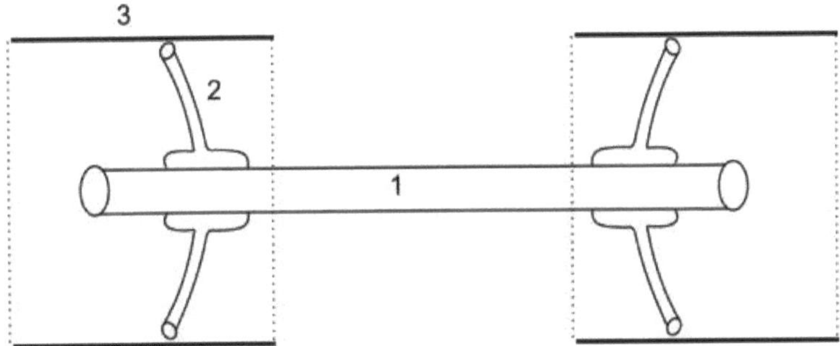

This figure shows the structure of the myofilament (the structural and functional unit of the myofibril), which consists of a single thick myosin fibre (1), around which are six thin actin fibres (3) connected by a myosin cross-bridge (2).

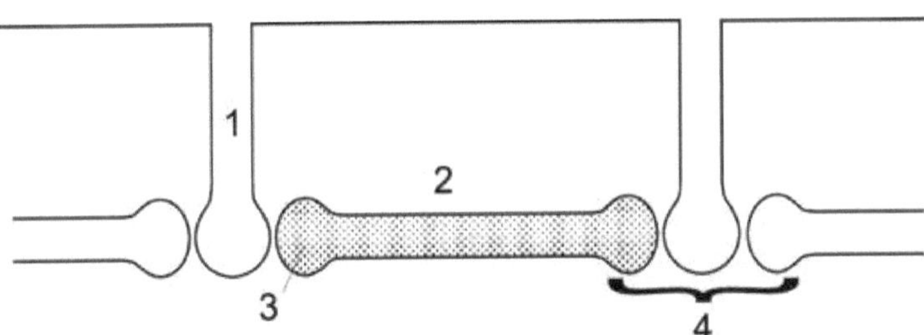

The scheme shows the structure of the T systems of a muscle fibre (4), which consists of one longitudinal tubule (1) and two transverse tubules (2). An MPD peak extends across the membrane of the longitudinal tubule. The transverse tubules contain calcium ions, therefore they are called calcium cisternae.

Interaction of myosin with actin

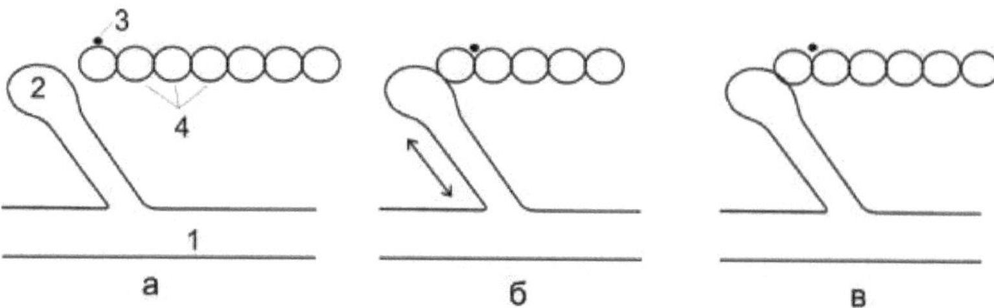

This diagram shows the mutual arrangement of the cross-bridge head (2) of myosin (1) and actin globules (4) in different states of the muscle: 1) relaxation (a), when the cross-bridge head is not connected to actin; 2) contraction (b), when the cross-bridge head is connected to actin and periodically ruptures, which promotes the sliding of actin along myosin (muscle contraction occurs); 3) rigor, or rigor mortis (c), when persistent attachment of the cross-bridge head to actin is noted.

Law of contraction of skeletal muscle and myocardium

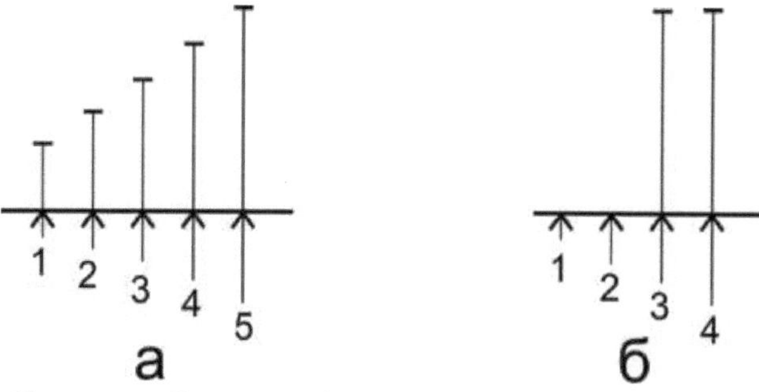

The diagram reflects two laws of muscle contraction: 1) the law of force (a) - the greater the strength of the stimulus (1-5), the greater the magnitude of the response; 2) the law of "all or nothing" (b) - the muscle either does not respond to the stimulus (1,2 - nothing), or responds with maximum reaction (3,4 -

everything). The law of force is noted in skeletal muscles. A muscle fibre is made up of many myofibrils, each of which is separate from each other and has its own excitability. When a threshold stimulus is applied, myofibrils with the highest excitability react. As the stimulus strength increases, the number of myofibrils involved in contraction increases, resulting in an increased response. The all-or-nothing law is characteristic of myocardium, whose cardiomyocytes are connected to each other by means of nexuses. At a certain stimulus strength, all cardiomyocytes are excited and the maximum response (all) occurs. The myocardium does not react to previous stimulus strengths (nothing).

PROPERTIES OF NERVES. MYONEURAL SYNAPSE

The structure of nerves

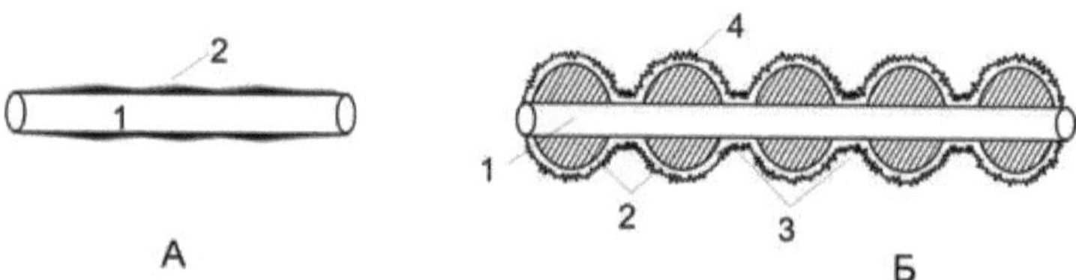

All nerves (the aggregate of the outgrowths of a neuron) are divided into two groups according to their structure: 1) unmyelinated nerves, or myelin-free nerves (A); 2) myelinated nerves (B), or fleshy nerves. Myelin-free nerves consist of an axial cylinder (1 - a collection of outgrowths) and the Schwann sheath (2). Myelinated nerves consist of: 1) axial cylinder (1); 2) myelin (2) - a lipid that acts as an insulator and also participates in mediator synthesis; 3) Ranvier intercepts (3) - a section of the nerve not covered by myelin; 4) Schwann sheath (4).

Mechanism of excitation transmission along the nerves

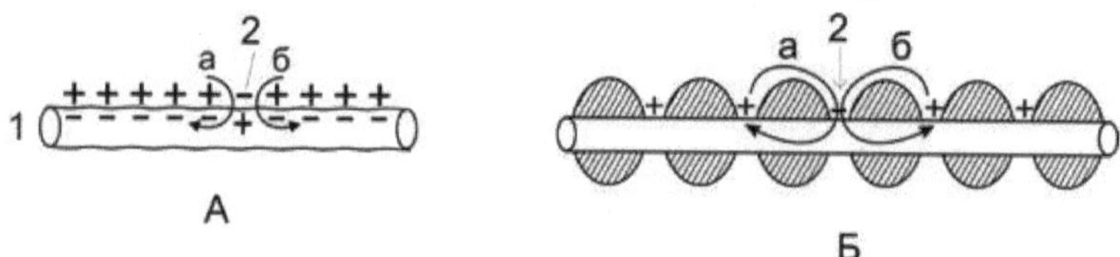

The diagram shows the mechanism of excitation transmission in myelinated (B) and unmyelinated nerves. When a stimulus is applied to a myelin-free nerve (A2), membrane depolarisation occurs, resulting in local currents (a,b) and membrane depolarisation of neighbouring areas on the left and right, excitation spreads in both directions (bilateral spread of excitation). In this case, excitation spreads over the entire membrane surface, so the speed of excitation transmission in unmyelinated nerves is very low (0.5 - 10 m/s). When a stimulus is applied to a myelinated nerve (B2), membrane depolarisation occurs, resulting in circular currents (a,b) between the Ranvier intercepts on the left and right and depolarisation of the membrane of these intercepts, excitation spreads in both directions (bilateral spread of excitation). In this case, excitation propagates from one Ranvier intercept to another or immediately to a third, so the speed of excitation transmission in myelinated nerves is very high (up to 70-120 m/s).

The laws of excitation in the nerves

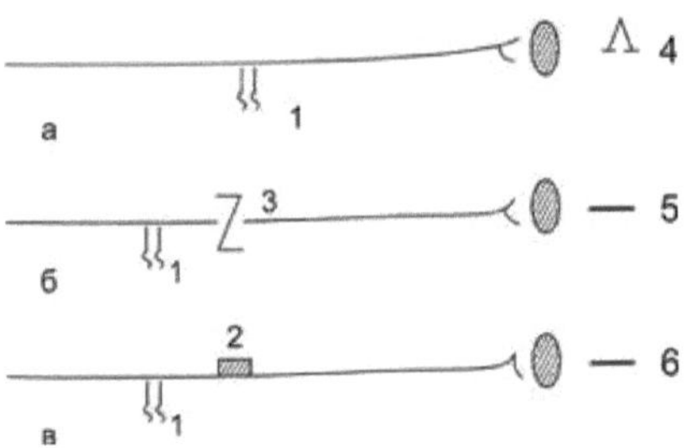

The diagram reflects one of the laws of nerve conduction: physiological and anatomical integrity of the nerve. Diagram a shows the anatomical and physiological integrity of a nerve. When this nerve is irritated (1), a response occurs (4). If anatomical (b) or physiological (c) integrity is compromised, irritation of the nerve (1b, 1c) does not elicit a response (5, 6).

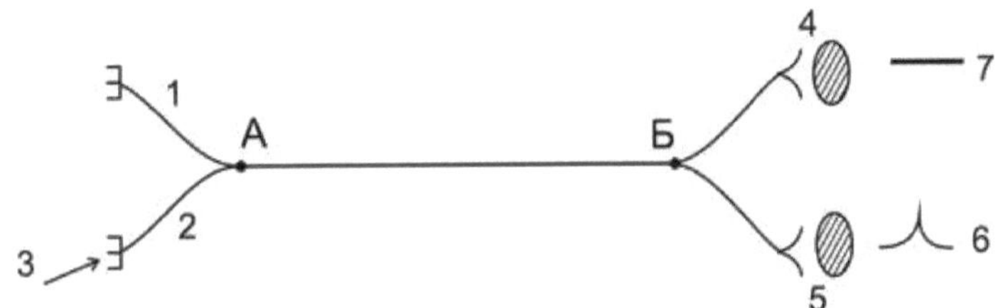

The diagram reflects the law of isolated conduction of excitation along a nerve. Efferent nerves 1 and 2 respectively terminate at effectors 4 and 5. Throughout A-B efferent nerves 1 and 2 go side by side. When receptor 3 is irritated, impulses along the efferent nerve go to effector 5 and the muscle contracts (6). Impulses from efferent nerve 2 in the A-B section do not pass to efferent nerve 1, so effector 4 does not respond to stimulation of receptor 3.

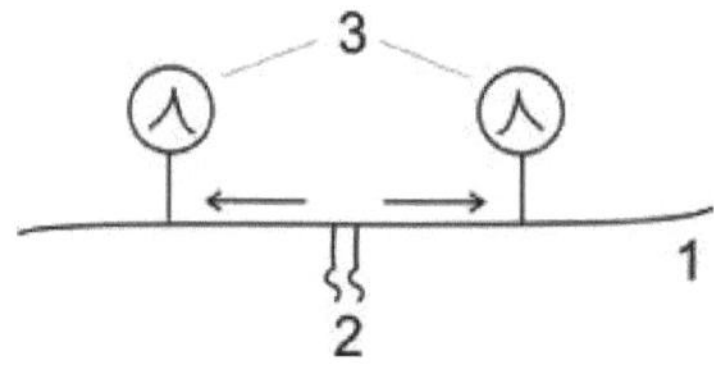

This diagram reflects the law of two-way conduction of excitation along the nerve. When a nerve is irritated (2), impulses flow in two directions, as evidenced by the registration of the membrane action potential (3) to the left and right of the site of irritation

Myoneural synapse. VPSP. TPSP

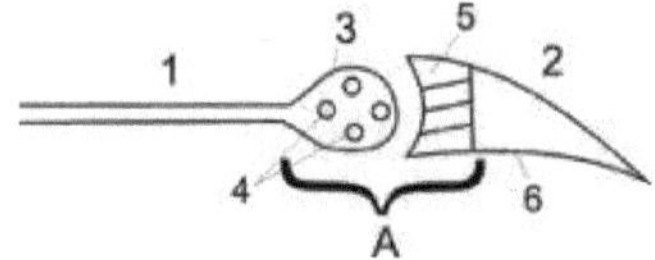

This diagram shows the structure of the myo-neural synapse (A), through which excitation is transmitted from the nerve (1) to the muscle (2). The myoneural synapse consists of: 1)presynaptic membrane (3), which contains vesicles (4) filled with physiologically active substance (mediator); 2) postsynaptic membrane (5), which differs from the extrasynaptic membrane (6) by the presence of a reactive substance that is highly sensitive to the mediator; 3)synaptic gap between the presynaptic and postsynaptic membrane. Through the synaptic cleft, excitation is transmitted chemically by mediator. The impulse (peak MAP) along the nerve reaches the presynaptic membrane, vesicles burst and mediator is released, which diffuses into the synaptic cleft and interacts with the reactive substance of the postsynaptic membrane. When the excitatory mediator is released, depolarisation occurs in the postsynaptic membrane and an excitatory postsynaptic potential (EPSP) is generated. If the PPSP reaches a critical level in the extrasynaptic membrane, a peak MAP occurs and spreads across the muscle membrane. When an inhibitory mediator is released in the postsynaptic membrane, hyperpolarisation occurs and an inhibitory postsynaptic potential (IPP) is generated and inhibition occurs.

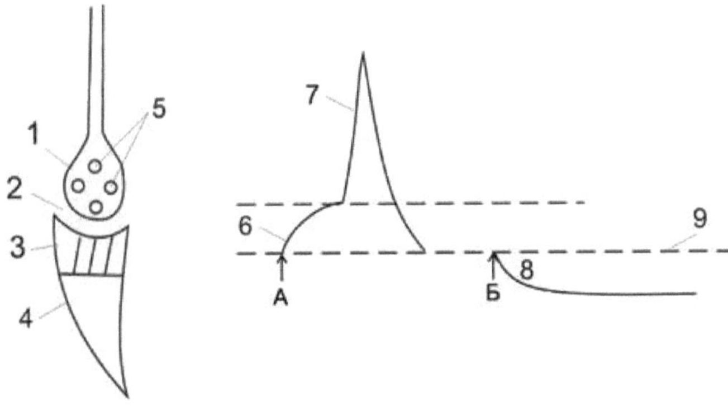

The diagram shows the mechanism of excitatory postsynaptic potential (EPSP - 6) and inhibitory postsynaptic potential (IPSP - 8). In the postsynaptic membrane (3) of myoneural synapses (1-3) can occur EPSP or TPSP, which depends on the mediator, which is located in vesicles (5) of the presynaptic membrane (1). When an excitatory mediator is released in the postsynaptic membrane (A), depolarisation occurs and a VPSP is formed. If the ERPP reaches a critical level in the extrasynaptic membrane (4), a peak MAP (7) occurs and spreads throughout the muscle membrane. When an inhibitory mediator is released, hyperpolarisation occurs in the postsynaptic membrane (B) and TPSP is formed and inhibition occurs. Thus, when a mediator acts on the postsynaptic membrane, its MPP (9) either decreases (depolarisation - when an excitatory mediator acts) or increases (hyperpolarisation - when an inhibitory mediator acts).

AUTONOMIC NERVOUS SYSTEM (ANS)

Peculiarities of the ANS and somatic nervous system divisions

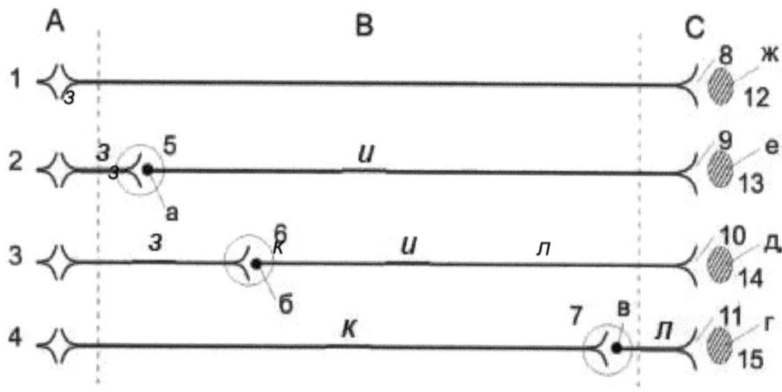

The diagram shows various neurons (A), their efferent nerves (B) with corresponding effectors (C). The somatic neuron (1) is localised in the anterior horns of the spinal cord. Its efferent nerve (somatic), without interruption, reaches the effector (g - sacetylcholine (8), which interacts with the H-choline-reactive substance of the postsynaptic membrane, resulting in an excitatory postsynaptic potential. The sympathetic neuron of the autonomic nervous system (2, 3) is localised in the lateral horns of the spinal cord of the cervical, thoracic and lumbar segments. Its efferent nerve terminates in the sympathetic ganglion (5,6), which is closer to the CNS. The efferent sympathetic nerve consists of pre (h) and postganglionic (i) fibres. The endings of the preganglionic fibre (sympathetic ganglion) release acetylcholine and the endings of the postganglionic fibre release norepinephrine. The postsynaptic membrane of the sympathetic ganglion (a,b) contains the H-choline-reactive substance. The postsynaptic membrane of the effector contains either alpha, beta1 or beta2 adrenergic substance, so either excitation of the effector (due to the interaction of norepinephrine with alpha or beta1 adrenergic substance) or inhibition (due to the interaction of norepinephrine with beta2 adrenergic substance) can occur here. Parasympathetic neurons (4) are localised: 1) in the lateral horns of the spinal cord of the sacral segments; 2) medulla oblongata; 3) midbrain. Its efferent nerve is terminated in the parasympathetic ganglion (7), which is closer to the working organ (effector). The efferent parasympathetic nerve consists of pre (k) and postganglionic (l) fibres. Acetylcholine is released at the endings of the preganglionic fibre (parasympathetic ganglion) and postganglionic fibre. The postsynaptic membrane of the parasympathetic ganglion (c) contains the H-choline-reactive substance. The postsynaptic membrane of the effector contains either H- or M-choline-reactive substance, so either excitation of the effector (by interaction of acetylcholine with H-choline-reactive substance) or inhibition (by interaction of acetylcholine with M-choline-reactive substance) can occur here.

Types of interaction between ANS divisions

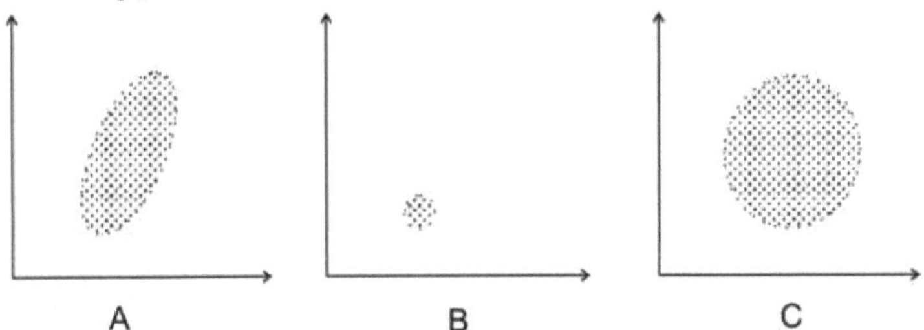

This figure shows the types of interaction between the departments of the autonomous nervous system (sympathetic and parasympathetic), determined by correlation rhythmograms (CRG): 1) normotonic type of interaction (A), when there is coordination (consistency) in the action of the departments of the autonomous nervous system (ANS) on the effector; 2)

sympathicotonic type of interaction (B), when there is discoordination (violation of consistency) in the action of the ANS departments on the effector with the prevailing influence of the sympathetic department; 3) vagotonic type of interaction (C), when there is discoordination (violation of coherence) in the action of ANS departments on the effector with the prevailing influence of the parasympathetic department.

CENTRAL NERVOUS SYSTEM (CNS)
The main neurons of the CNS

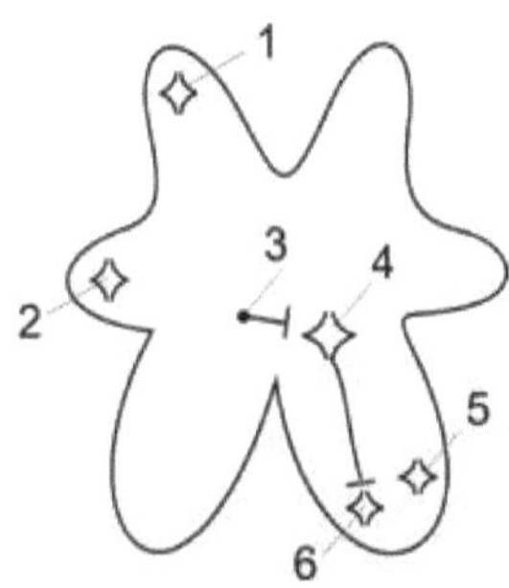

The figure shows a transverse section of the spinal cord (grey matter) with localisation of the main neurons: 1 - afferent neurons (sensitive), localised in the posterior horns; 2 - autonomic neurons, localised in the lateral horns, whose branches form sympathetic and parasympathetic nerves; 3 - inhibitory interneurons, the excitation of which results in the inhibition of Renshaw's giant inhibitory cells (4), resulting in the facilitation of spinal reflexes; 4 - Renshaw's giant inhibitory cells, the excitation of which results in the inhibition of the alpha motoneurons of the anterior horns (6), resulting in the inhibition of spinal reflexes; 5 - gamma motoneurons, whose outgrowths end in the intrafusal muscles. When these neurons are excited, intrafusal muscles contract and the tone of extrafusal (skeletal) muscles increases; 6 - alpha motoneurons of the anterior horns, whose outgrowths end in extrafusal muscles. When these neurons are excited, the tone of skeletal muscles increases.

Peculiarities of excitation conduction in the CNS

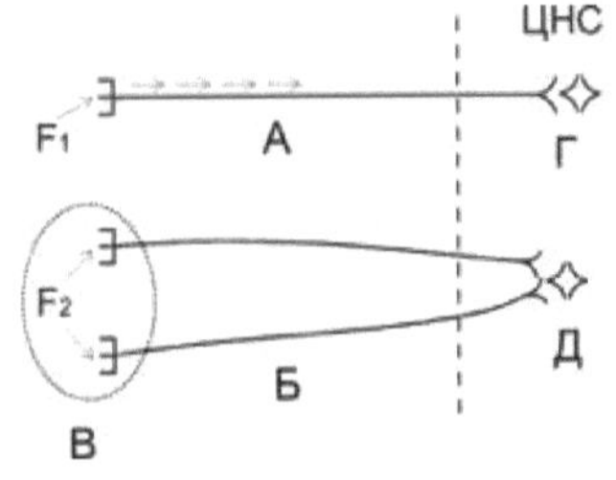

This figure reflects one of the features of excitation conduction in the central nervous system (CNS) - summation of excitation. Two types of summation are distinguished: 1) sequential or temporal summation (A), which occurs during the action of a rhythmic stimulus of a certain frequency (F1). In this case in the CNS there is a summation of the released mediator in the presynaptic membrane. At a very small frequency (1-5 Hz) of the stimulus, summation does not occur, because before the next impulse arrives, the mediator from the previous impulse diffuses into the synaptic cleft and is destroyed; 2) spatial or simultaneous summation (B), which occurs when a single or rhythmic stimulus (F2) acts simultaneously on two or more receptors of the same receptive field (a set of receptors whose irritation produces the same reaction). In this case, mediator summation in the synaptic cleft occurs.

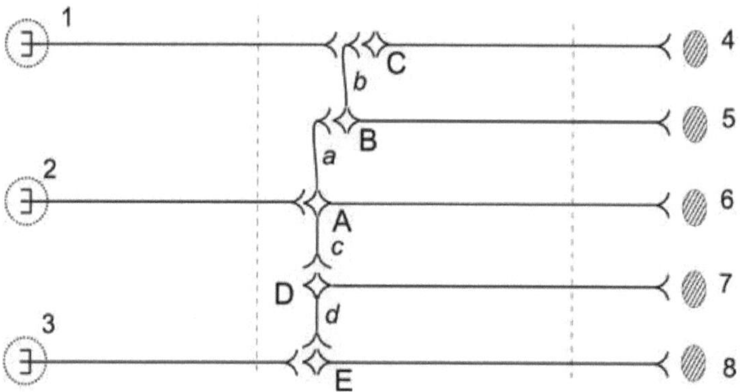

This diagram shows one of the features of excitation conduction in the CNS - excitation irradiation, the spread of excitation in the CNS from one neuron (A) to other neurons (B,C,D,E) and even to those neurons that do not belong to the given receptive field (2). At threshold and submaximal stimulation of receptors 1, 2, 3, respectively, neurons C, A, E are excited and effectors 4, 6, and 8 respond. When maximum and supramaximal stimulus is applied to receptor 3, not only neuron A, but also neurons B, C, D, and E are excited through outgrowths a, c, d, e, i.e. excitation is irradiated in the CNS through numerous insertion neurons.

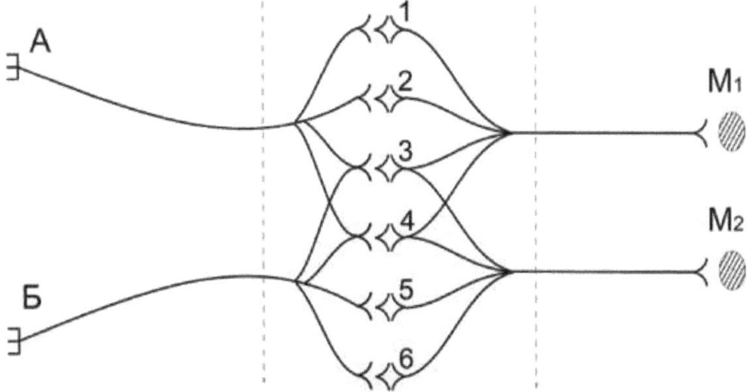

This scheme reflects one of the peculiarities of excitation conduction in the CNS - occlusion, i.e. blockage. When each receptor (A, B) is irritated separately, 4 neurons are excited in the CNS: neurons 1,2,3,4 are excited when receptor A is irritated, and neurons 3,4,5,6 are excited when receptor B is irritated. This diagram shows that neurons 3 and 4 in the CNS are common to receptors A and B. During simultaneous stimulation, 6 neurons in the CNS are excited instead of 8 neurons. Neurons 3 and 4 are excited by a competitive mechanism either by stimulation of receptor A or by stimulation of receptor B. If neurons 3,4 are excited by impulses arising from stimulation of receptor A, then for a certain time these neurons will be in the refractory phase of excitability and will not respond to impulses arising from stimulation of receptor B and vice versa. Thus, as a result of occlusion (blockage of impulses arising from stimulation of receptor A or B) when receptors A and B are stimulated simultaneously, the response of effectors M1 and M2 will be less than the sum of the response of each effector when each receptor is stimulated separately.

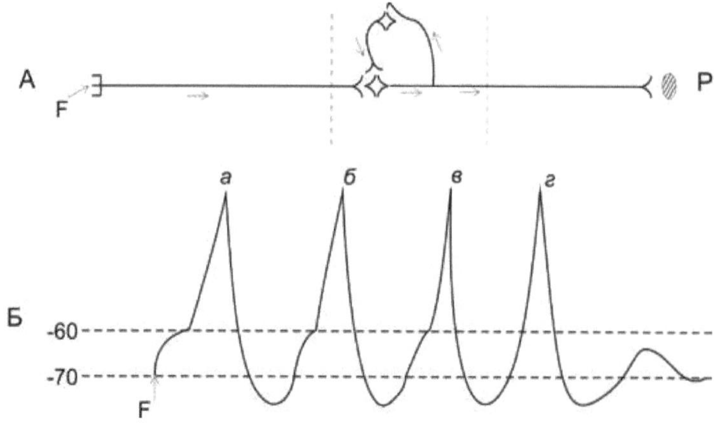

This diagram reflects one of the features of excitation conduction in the CNS - aftereffect, i.e. preservation of excitation in the CNS after cessation of stimulus action. There are short-term (B) and long-term (A) aftereffects. Prolonged aftereffect (A) occurs on the action of maximum or supermaximal stimulus (F). In this case, there is a prolonged circulation of the impulse in the CNS, through the insertion excitatory neuron, so that at a single stimulus of the receptor in the CNS excitation is preserved for a long time and there is a prolonged response of the effector (P) after the cessation of stimulation of the receptor. A short-term aftereffect (B) can occur when a threshold stimulus (F) is applied. This is due to the peculiarity of MFM occurrence in neurons and low threshold stimulus: the difference between MFP (-70 mv) and critical level of depolarisation (-60 mv). When MPP occurs in neurons, there is a high level of trace depolarisation (d, d1, d2), so a single stimulus causes 4 reactions: reaction a in response to the stimulus, responses b, c, d are aftereffects - a reaction to a high level of trace depolarisation.

Presynaptic inhibition (localisation and mechanism)

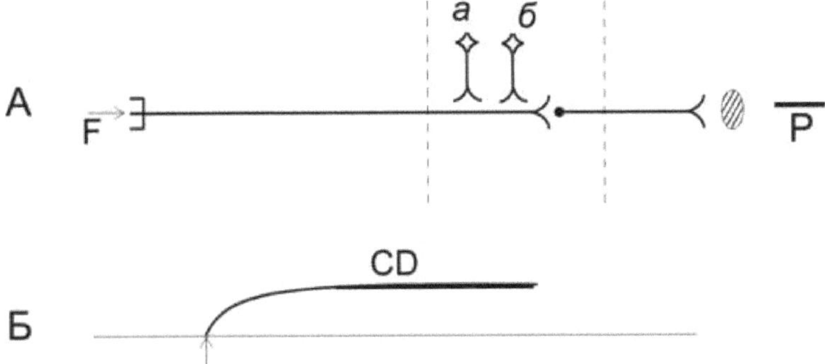

This scheme reflects one of the types of inhibition in the CNS (A) - presynaptic (T), which arises as a result of constant weak excitation of insertion neurons a, b, impulses from which come to the presynaptic terminal, where persistent depolarisation occurs (B - CD). In this case, sodium channels are blocked in the presynaptic terminal, as a result of which impulses arising from receptor stimulation (F) do not pass through T, no mediator is released in the presynaptic membrane (1), and there is no effector response (P).

Types of postsynaptic inhibition

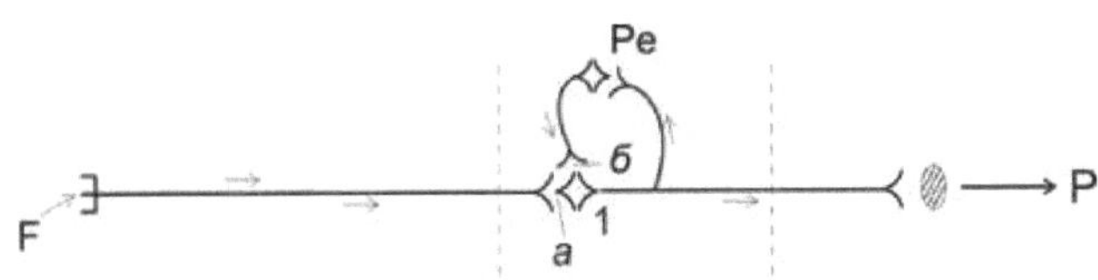

This diagram reflects one of the types of postsynaptic inhibition in the CNS - return inhibition. When a receptor (F) is strongly stimulated, impulses go not only to the effector (E), but also return to the neuron (1) via Renshaw cells (Re) via collaterals, causing its hyperpolarisation (inhibition).

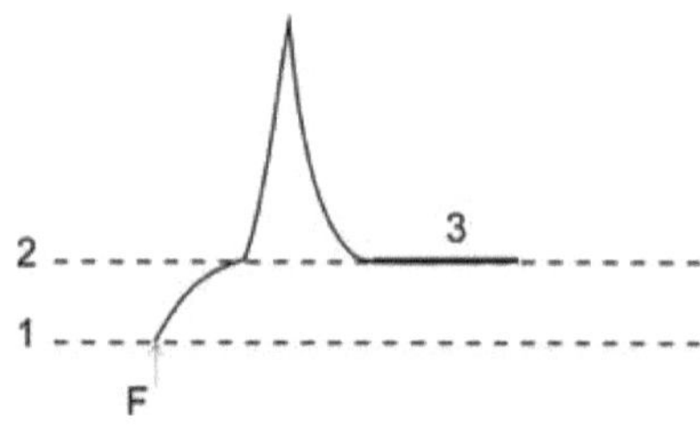

This diagram shows one of the types of postsynaptic inhibition - pessimal inhibition, which occurs under the action of a rhythmic stimulus of high frequency. The mechanism of this inhibition is based on persistent depolarisation, which is caused by the high frequency of the stimulus, as a result of which the mediator from the previous stimulus does not have time to be destroyed - repolarisation does not reach the level of polarisation (1), but remains at the level of critical depolarisation (2) for a long time - persistent depolarisation of the membrane occurs (3). In this case, blocking of sodium channels occurs, due to which the membrane does not respond to the action of any stimulus.

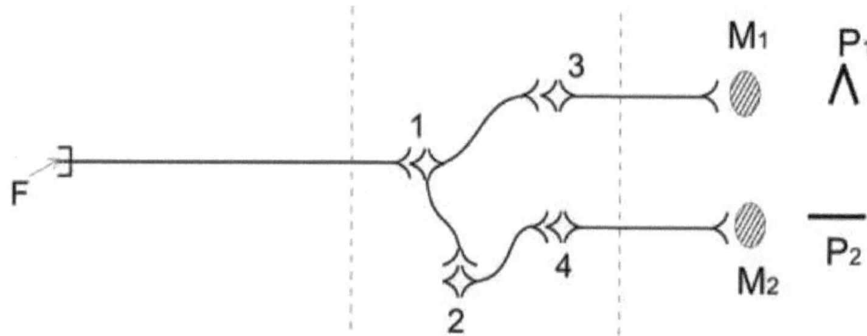

This diagram reflects one of the types of inhibition in the CNS - reciprocal or conjugate inhibition. When a stimulus (F) acts on a receptor, an afferent neuron (1) is excited. Impulses from this neuron go in two directions: directly to the alpha motoneuron (3) and through the giant inhibitory cells of Renshaw (2) to another alpha motoneuron. This results in an excitatory postsynaptic potential (EPSP) in the postsynaptic membrane of the first motoneuron (3) and further excitation is transmitted to the muscle (M1), which contracts (P1). In the postsynaptic membrane of the second alpha motoneuron (4) an inhibitory postsynaptic potential (IPSP) occurs, inhibition occurs and the muscle (M2) does not contract. The cause of PPSP is the mediator GABA (gamma aminobutyric acid), which increases the permeability to potassium ions, resulting in hyperpolarisation of the postsynaptic membrane.

This scheme reflects one of the types of inhibition in the CNS - Sechenov inhibition. After dissecting the optic tubercles (2) in the frog, we check the time of the reflex. For this purpose we apply irritation (with sulphuric acid solution - F) to the receptor (6). At the same time impulses through afferent neuron (7) arrive to alpha motoneuron (4), in the postsynaptic membrane of which there is an EPSP and excitation is further transferred to the muscle (5), there is a response (pulling of the foot - reflex). We determine the reflex time (time from the moment of stimulation to the appearance of a response). After that we apply salt crystals (1) to the optic tubercles (2). The resulting impulses, via inhibitory Renshaw cells, enter the postsynaptic membrane of the alpha motoneuron (4). In the presynaptic membrane of the Renshaw cell outgrowth, GABA is released, causing hyperpolarisation of the postsynaptic membrane of the alpha motoneuron (4), leading to a decrease in excitability. As a result, when the previous stimulus is applied to the receptor (6), it takes more time for a response to occur - inhibition occurs.

Principle of finite paths and re-capability

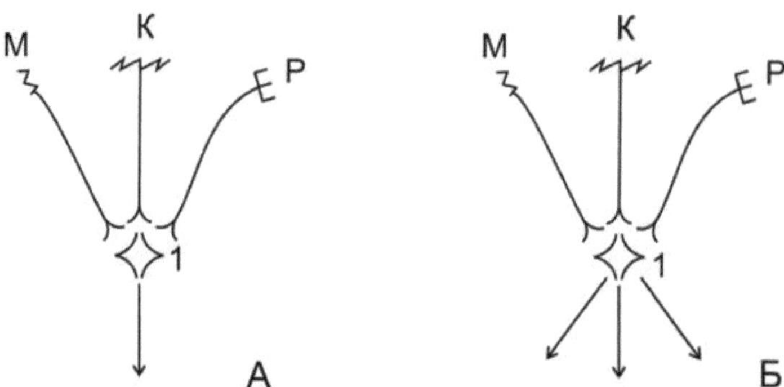

This diagram reflects one of the principles of CNS coordination activity - the principle of the final pathway. The alpha motoneuron (1) simultaneously receives impulses from the cerebellum (M), the cerebellar cortex (K) and the receptor (P). The choice of the final pathway can be made in two ways: 1) by the competitive principle (A), i.e. one response occurs, the most important one by inhibition of others; 2) by the allied mechanism (B), i.e. all three responses are noted mutually reinforcing each other.

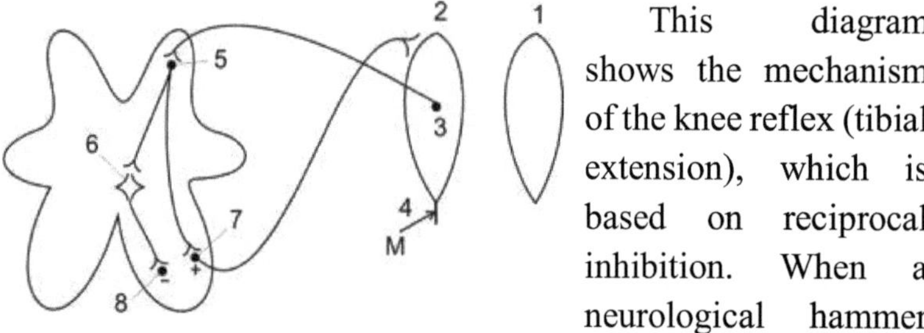

This diagram shows the mechanism of the knee reflex (tibial extension), which is based on reciprocal inhibition. When a neurological hammer (M) strikes the tendon of the tibial extensor muscle (4), this muscle (2) is stretched and the receptors of the muscle spindle (3) are excited. Impulses from this receptor via afferent neurons (5) simultaneously enter inhibitory Renshaw cells (6) and alpha motoneurons of the tibialis extensor muscles (7). Impulses from Renshaw cells go to the alpha motoneuron of the tibialis flexor muscles (8) and cause their inhibition, resulting in relaxation of this muscle. The alpha motoneuron of the tibialis extensor muscles (7) is excited and from here impulses go to the tibialis extensor muscles, causing their contraction. Thus, when a neurological hammer is struck on the tendon of the tibial extensor muscles, the alpha motoneurons of the tibial extensor muscles are simultaneously excited and the flexor muscles are relaxed - the tibial extensor (knee reflex) is observed

Tonic reflexes

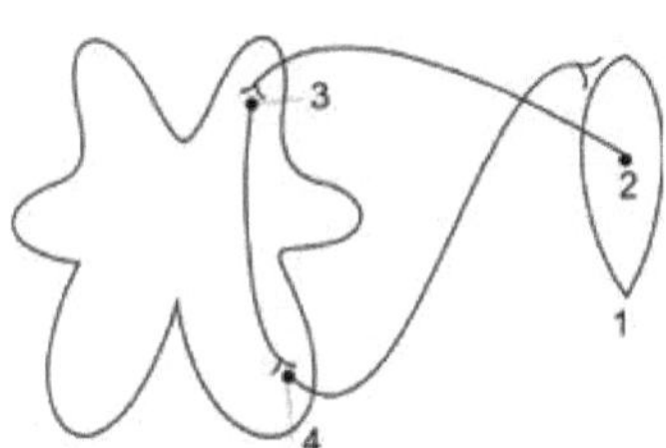

This diagram reflects the mechanism of the peripheral tonic reflex. When a muscle is relaxed (1), it is stretched, which leads to tension of the nuclear pouch of the muscle spindle (2). Impulses from this receptor via afferent neurons (3) go to alpha motoneurons (4) and from here to the muscle, causing its contraction (muscle tone increases).

This diagram shows the mechanism of central muscle tone. Upon excitation of reticular neurons (1), impulses along the reticulospinal pathway reach gamma motoneurons (2) in the anterior horns of the spinal

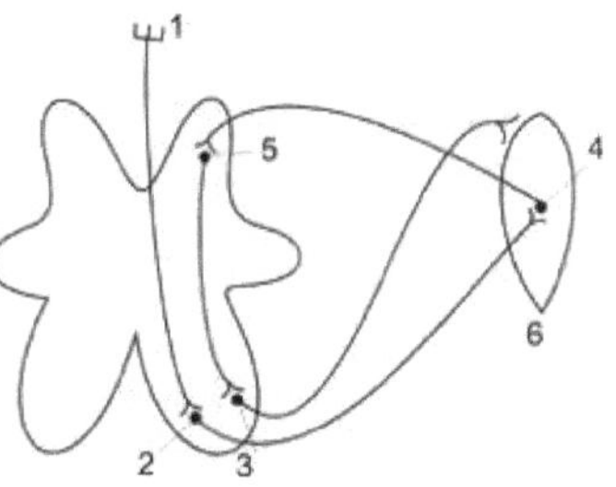

cord. From gamma motoneurones impulses go to the intrafusal muscles of the muscle spindle (4). When these muscles contract, the nuclear bag is stretched and excitation from the receptors of the nuclear bag through afferent neurons (5) reaches alpha motoneurons (3) of extrafusal muscles (6), these muscles contract and their tone increases.

Reticulo-spinal tracts

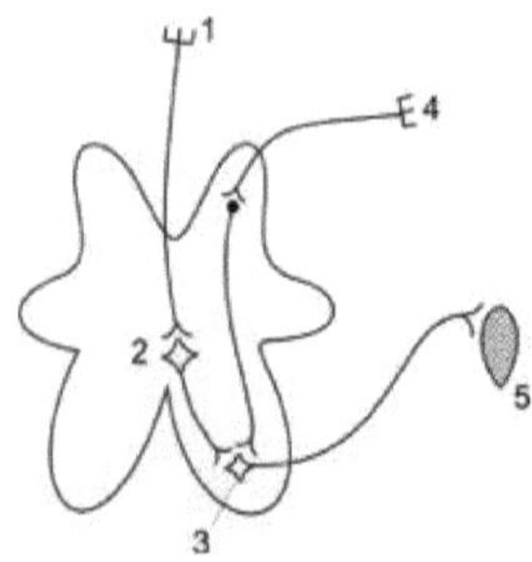

This diagram shows the reticulospinal pathway that causes inhibition of spinal reflexes. Impulses from the reticular formation via inhibitory Renshaw cells (2) arrive to the alpha motoneuron (3) of the skeletal muscle (5). This causes hyperpolarisation of the postsynaptic membrane of this neuron. As a result, when the receptor (4) is irritated, inhibition of this reflex occurs.

This diagram shows the reticulospinal pathway that facilitates spinal reflexes. Impulses from the reticular formation via inhibitory interneurons (2) arrive at inhibitory Renshaw cells (3), causing their inhibition. The release of gamma aminobutyric acid (GABA) stops (or decreases) in the presynaptic membrane of the outgrowth of Renshaw cells, which leads to an increase in the excitability of the alpha motoneuron, facilitating spinal reflexes.

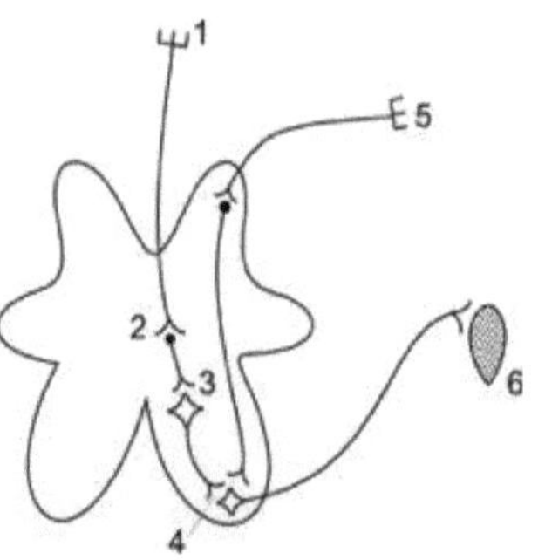

Interaction of the PMA, Hess centre and reticular formation

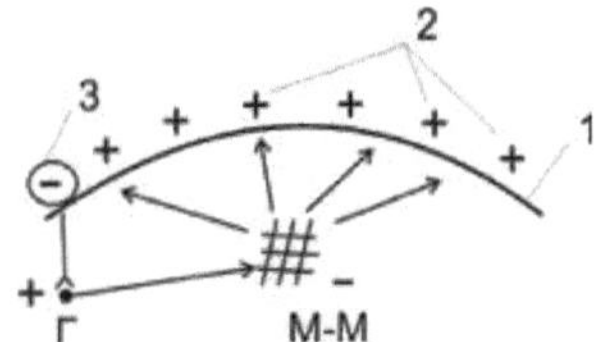

This diagram shows the interaction between the cerebral cortex (PMA-1), the Magune Morutsi centre of the brain reticular formation (M-M) and the Hess centre in the hypothalamus (H). When the Hess centre is excited, the Magoon Moruci centre is inhibited and the flow of impulses through the reticulocortical pathway stops, which leads to inhibition of the PMA (1). Thus, in the awake state, the Magoon Moruci centre is in the state of excitation. Due to impulses along the reticulocortical pathway, the PMA is in an active state (2). When local inhibition occurs in the PMA (3), the Hess centre is excited, which leads to inhibition of the Meguna Moruci centre, the flow of impulses along the reticulocortical pathway stops, and the PMA is inhibited (sleep occurs).

PHYSIOLOGICAL REGULATION

Somatic and autonomic reflex arcs

This diagram shows somatic (B) and autonomic (A) reflex pathways. The somatic reflex pathway begins with the receptor (1), where the energy of the stimulus is converted into a 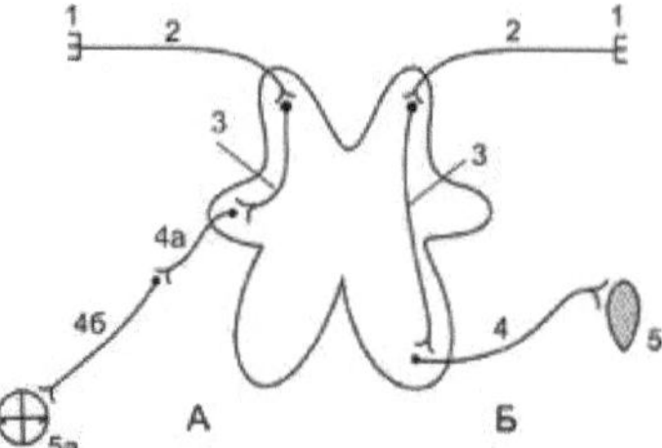 nerve impulse, which reaches the anterior horns of the spinal cord via the afferent neuron along the afferent pathway (2). From here, impulses along the efferent pathway (4) reach the working organ, the skeletal muscles (5). The autonomic reflex pathway begins with the receptor (1), where the energy of the stimulus is converted into a nerve impulse, which reaches the lateral horns of the spinal cord via the afferent neuron along the afferent pathway (2). From here, impulses along the efferent pathway (4) reach the working organ, the internal organs (in this case the myocardium - 5a). The efferent pathway of the autonomic reflex pathway is interrupted in the ganglion and consists of pre- (4a) and postganglionic fibres (4b). Thus, the somatic and autonomic reflex pathway consists of 5 links: receptor (1), afferent pathway (2), insertion neuron (3), efferent pathway (4, 4a, 4b) and effector (working organ - 5, 5a)

Feedback principle

1

This diagram shows the nerve regulation of physiological functions with feedback. Nervous regulation begins

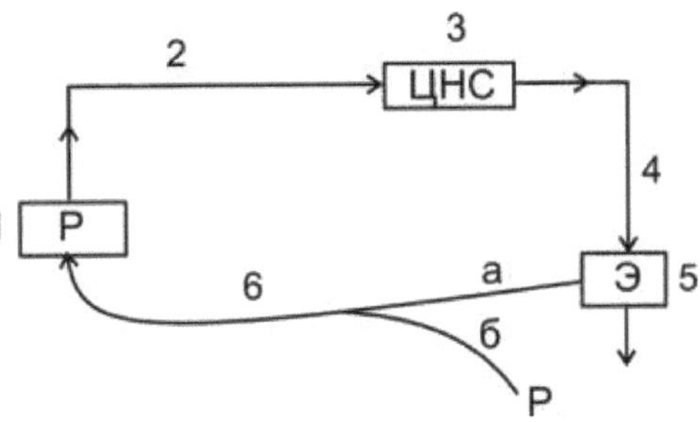

with receptor irritation (1 - P). Impulses from the receptor along the afferent pathway (2) arrive to the CNS (3), then along the efferent pathways (4) to the effector (5 - E), and the result (P1) appears. The result of the effector via feedback (6) enters the CNS from either the effector receptors (a) or the receptor perceiving the result (b). Thus, the feedback carries information to the CNS about the actual result. Here the actual result is compared with the set (proper) result. If the actual result is greater than the target result, the effector function decreases (negative feedback), if the actual result is less than the target result, the effector function increases (positive feedback).

This diagram reflects the signals affecting the effector (Ef). All signals are divided into two groups: 1 - setting signals coming from the CNS; 2 - perturbing signals,

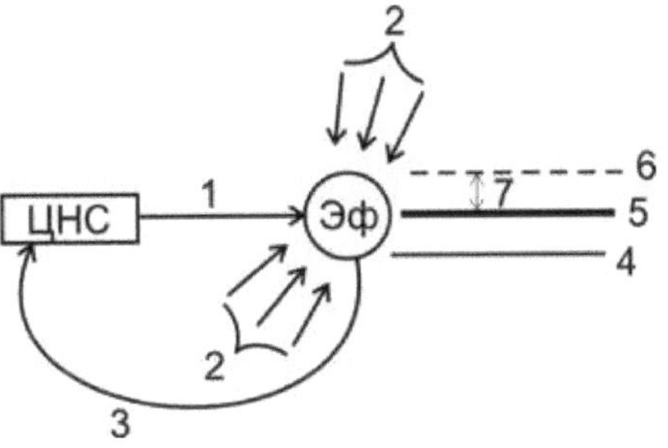

their number depends on the environment in which the person is. Setting signals set the effector's operation to a preset level (5). Perturbing signals deviate the effector's work from the set level (6,4), so the actual result of the effector's work always differs from the set one. The difference between the parameters of the set result and the actual result (7) indicates a mismatch. Thanks to feedback (3), the mismatch is minimised.

Peculiarities of nervous and humoral regulation

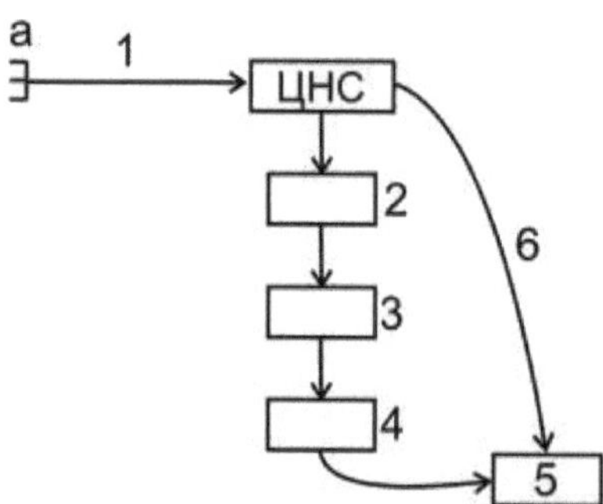

This diagram shows the nervous (a-1-CNS-6-5) and humoral (a-1-CNS-2-3-4-5) regulation of physiological functions. At nervous regulation impulses from the receptor (a) through afferent pathways (1) arrive to the CNS, from where they go to the effector (5) through efferent pathways (6). Nervous regulation is carried out on the basis of reflexes. In humoral regulation impulses from the receptor (a) through afferent pathways (1) arrive in the CNS. This excites the hypothalamus (2), resulting in the release of liberins or statins, which through the autonomous portal system arrive in the anterior lobe of the pituitary gland - adenohypophysis (3). Here, the release of the corresponding tropic hormone is either increased (by the action of liberins) or decreased (by the action of statins). The tropic hormones of the pituitary gland through the blood affect the corresponding endocrine glands (4), which secrete an effector hormone that affects the function of the effector through the blood (5). Thus, in humoral regulation, several intermediate effectors (2,3,4) are involved in the process, so the speed of humoral regulation is much slower than that of nervous regulation.

Functional body systems (FBS)

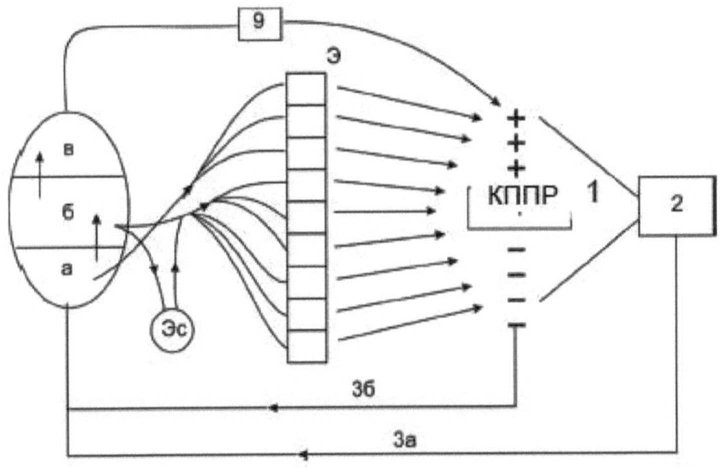

This diagram shows the links of the functional system of the organism (FUS). According to P.K. Anokhin's definition, a FUS is a dynamic organisation, the activity of which is aimed at achieving some final useful adaptive result (1 - KPPP). Thus, the system-forming factor of any FUS is KPPR. It is a dynamic organisation, as the number of effectors involved in a particular QSF is constantly changing, and if the KPPR is within the norm, the QSF does not function. The first link of the QSF is the CPPR. When the CPPP deviates from the optimal level, the second link, the specific receptor (2), is excited. From the specific receptor impulses via afferent pathway (3a) arrive to the CNS. In addition, the change of the index itself, through the humoral link (3b), also affects the CNS. Three levels are distinguished in the CNS: a) the specific centre, which is excited by the change of any indicator; b) hypothalamus, which is the supreme centre of all vegetative and endocrine functions; c) the cortex of the large hemispheres, which, when excited, switches on the external link of the FUS - purposeful behaviour aimed at a specific result. From the specific centre and the hypothalamus through efferent pathways impulses arrive at the effectors, the work of which changes this CPPP. When the hypothalamus is involved in the process, in parallel with nerve impulses, the humoral link of influence on the effectors through changes in the functions of endocrine glands is included. The number of effectors participating in the work of the FUS depends on the degree of deviation of the CPPP from the optimal level: the greater the deviation, the more effectors participate in the work of this FUS. If at maximum change of the effectors' functions, the CPPP is not restored to normal, excitation from the hypothalamus spreads to the cortex of the large hemispheres and an external link - behaviour - is included in the work of the FUS. Behaviour will change one by one until the CPPP is restored to the optimal value.

Central link of the QSF

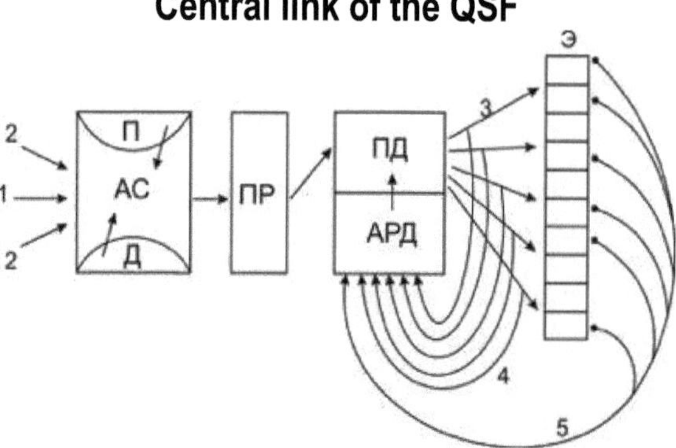

This scheme reflects the central link of the FUS, which consists of the following blocks: I. Afferent synthesis (AS), where signals of several orders are combined: a) trigger signal (1), which comes from a specific receptor and indicates a deviation of the CPPD; b) situational signals (2), which carry information about the environment in which the object is located through the appropriate receptors; c) signals from the memory unit (M); d) signals from the dominant focus of excitation (E). When the above signals are combined, the AS answers the following questions: 1) what to do? When combining trigger and circumstance signals; 2) how to do? When combining the trigger, status signals and those coming from the memory block; 3) when to do? When combining the trigger, circumstance signals from the memory unit and the dominant arousal focus; II. Decision making (DP); III. Programmes of action (PoA), i.e. which effectors (E) and in what mode should function to return the CPPP to the optimal level; IV. When realising the PD (3), the fourth block is formed (4) - the action result acceptor (ARD) - this block P.K. Anokhin called the apparatus of future foresight. This block reflects the parameters of the future functioning of effectors, i.e. what the parameters of effector functioning should be. When the function of the effectors changes, signals about their actual result are fed to the RDA by feedback (5). This block compares the set result (via PD) with the actual result received via feedback. If the actual result does not coincide with the set result, the pulses from the ADF go to the PD and the already functioning effectors are changed.

CARDIOVASCULAR SYSTEM

Recording of cardiac action potentials
(EKG, Einthoven's triangle)

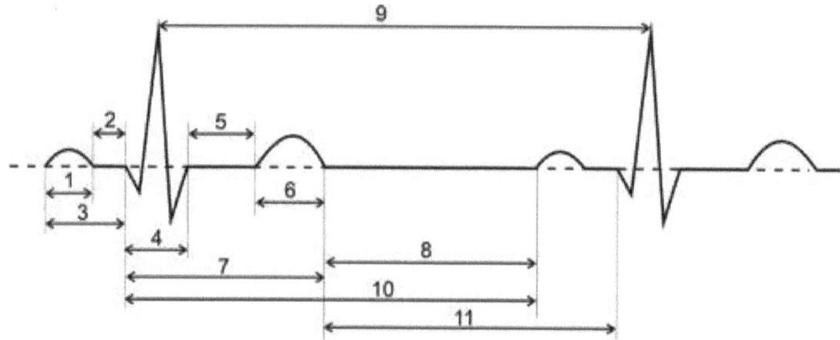

ECG. The following intervals are marked here: PQ (3) - time of excitation propagation from atria to ventricles; QRS (4) - time of excitation propagation through myocardium of both ventricles; QRST (7) - time during which the presence of excitation process in heart ventricles is noted - duration of electrical systole; RR (9) - duration of one cardiac cycle (systole and diastole). On ECG we distinguish the following segments (the part of the interval that is on the isoline); PQ (2) - the part of the PQ interval that is on the isoline. This segment reflects the process of polarisation, as excitation in the atria has ended and in the ventricles has not yet begun; ST (5) - the part of the interval QRST, which is on the isoline. This segment reflects the process of depolarisation - during this time all myocardial fibres are in a state of excitation; TP (8) - at this time myocardium is in a state of polarisation, as excitation in the ventricles has ended and atria has not started (myocardium of the ventricles and atria are at rest - general pause). Duration of P (1) - the time during which the excitation process is observed in both atria. Duration of T (6) - time of excitation decay (repolarisation) in the ventricles of the heart. 10 - duration of atrial diastole; 11 - duration of ventricular diastole.

Physiological properties of cardiac muscle.
Cardiac automatism

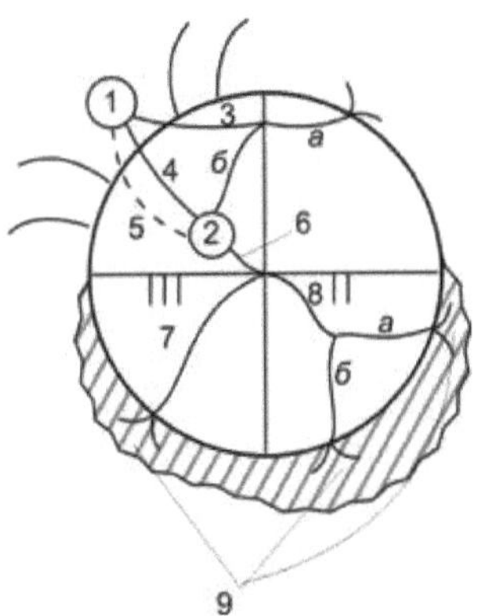

The conduction system of the heart, which consists of the following elements:

1) sinoatrial node (SA), located at the border of the venous sinus (the junction of the superior and inferior vena cava) and the right atrium. This node has the greatest automaticity; 2) atrioventricular node (AV), located on the interventricular septum closer to the interatrial septum. The automaticity of this node is 1.5 times less than that of the CA node. The CA node is connected to the AV by three inter-nodal bundles: anterior inter-nodal bundle (3), which divides into two branches one of which reaches the left atrium (3a - Bachmann's bundle), the other (3b) to the AV; middle inter-nodal bundle (4 - Wenckebach's bundle) starts from the SA, passes behind the superior vena cava, descends down the posterior part of the interatrial septum and reaches the AV; posterior inter-nodal bundle (5 - Thorel's bundle) leaves the SA goes downwards and posteriorly. The bundle of Hiss (6) - begins in the lower part of the AV and in the area of the interventricular septum divides into two legs: the right leg of the bundle of Hiss (7) - a long thin bundle, which in the distal part leaves the interventricular septum and reaches the anterior papillary muscle of the right ventricle, where it branches and connects with Purkinje fibres; the left leg of the bundle of Hiss (8), which divides into two branches - anterior and posterior. The anterior branch reaches the base of the anterior papillary muscle and branches in the anterior-upper part of the left ventricle. The posterior branch reaches the base of the posterior papillary muscle. The cardiac conduction system ends in the ventricular myocardium with Purkinje fibres (9)

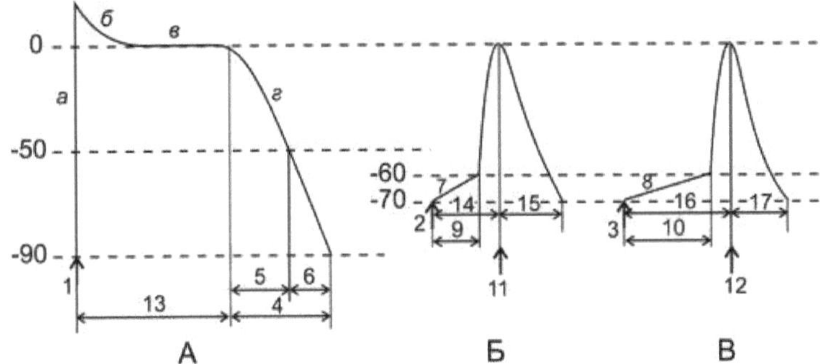

Figure A shows the MAP of a cardiomyocyte, which consists of the following phases: f. depolarisation (1), early, or fast, repolarisation (b), plateau (c), and late, or slow, repolarisation (d). The following phases of myocardial excitability correspond to the MAP phases: 1, b, c (13) corresponds to the absolute refractory phase, when the myocardium does not respond to additional stimuli. The duration of this phase corresponds to the duration of systole and the first third of diastole; d (5) corresponds to the relative refractory phase of excitability, in this phase the myocardium reacts to additional stimulation resulting in extrasystole; d (6) corresponds to the supernormal phase of excitability (exaltation).

Figure B shows the MAP in the sinoatrial node (SA) of the cardiac conduction system and consists of the following phases: slow diastolic depolarisation (SDD-9), which starts during ventricular diastole (2); depolarisation, which starts from the critical level of depolarisation (-60) and reaches the zero level, i.e., unlike the cardiomyocyte MAP, there is no overshoot; repolarisation, which starts from the zero level and reaches the -70 level.i.e., unlike cardiomyocyte MFD, there is no overshoot; repolarisation, which starts from the zero level and reaches the level of -70. At the onset of the MFD peak (11), an impulse in the SA occurs, to which the myocardium responds with the onset of systole. Thus, the duration from the onset of MFM (2) to peak MFM (11) corresponds to ventricular diastole (14). From the peak of MFM (11) to the beginning of the next MFM corresponds to ventricular systole (15).

Figure B shows the MAP in the atrioventricular node (AV) of the cardiac conduction system and consists of the following phases: slow diastolic depolarisation (MDD-10), which starts during ventricular diastole (3); depolarisation, which starts from the critical level of depolarisation (-60) and reaches the zero level, there is also no overhang; repolarisation, which starts from the zero level and reaches the -70 level. At the onset of the MAP peak (12), an impulse in AV occurs, to which the myocardium responds with the onset of systole. Thus, the duration from the onset of MFM (3) to peak MFM (12) corresponds to ventricular diastole (16). From the peak of MFM (12) to the beginning of the next MFM corresponds to ventricular systole (17).

Figures B and C show that MFM in the CA node differs from MFM in the AV node only by the different MFM rate: the MFM rate in the CA node (7) is greater than the MFM rate in the AV node (8); therefore, the automaticity of the CA node is significantly (1.5-2 times) higher than that of the AV node. In a healthy person, taking into account the influence of the vagus nerve on the heart, 60-80 impulses/min occur in 1min in the CA node, and 40-45 impulses/min in the AV node. When impulses occur in the SA node, impulses do not occur in the underlying parts of the conduction system (AV node, bundle of Hiss, legs of Hiss, Purkinje fibres) - they conduct impulses occurring in the SA node to the ventricular myocardium.

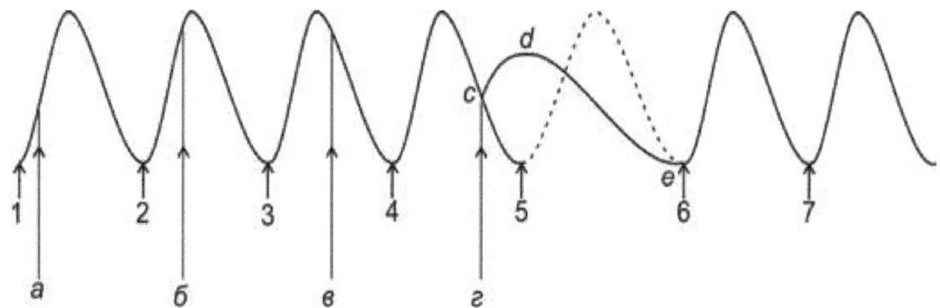

This figure shows the cardiogram and mechanism of cardiac ventricular extrasystole (c-d) followed by a compensatory pause, or prolonged diastole (d-e). 1-7 are impulses periodically occurring in the venous sinus (frog heart cardiogram); a-d are additional stimuli. The figure shows that of all the additional stimuli, the ventricular myocardium responds only to stimulus d (resulting in an extraordinary systole - extrasystole:c-d), which falls in the middle of diastole, which corresponds to the relative refractory phase. The ventricular myocardium does not respond to additional stimuli a,b,c, as these stimuli fall in the absolute refractory phase of excitability. After extrasystole there is a compensatory pause, or prolonged diastole (d-e), that is, after extrasystole one cardiac cycle (from imp. 5 to imp. 6) is skipped. The occurrence of d-e is due to the fact that the next impulse from the venous sinus (5) falls into the absolute refractory phase of myocardial excitability (extrasystole) and the myocardium does not respond to this stimulus until the next (6) impulse occurs.

Haemodynamic function of the heart. The structure of the cardiac cycle

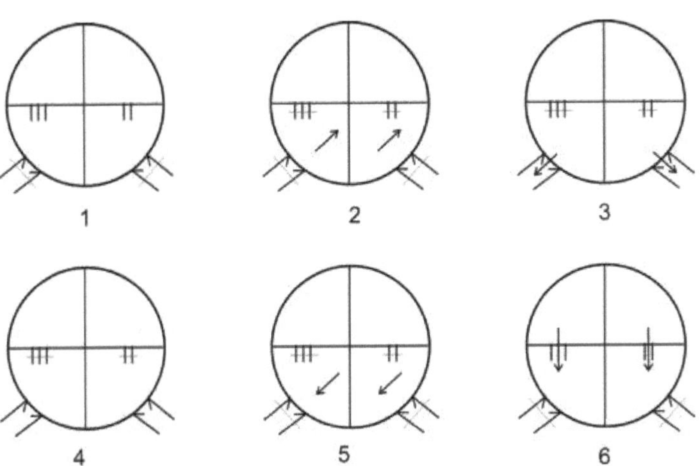

These figures show the correspondence of the flap valves (on the atrial-ventricular septum) and semilunar valves (at the mouth of the pulmonary artery from the right ventricle and aorta from the left ventricle) in different phases and periods of the cardiac cycle structure. In Fig.1, the flap valves are open and the semilunar valves are closed - this corresponds to the beginning of systole (period of asynchronous contraction - As), not all myocardial fibres of the ventricles have been excited yet, so the flap valves are still open. As lasts for 0.04-0.05s. In Fig. 2, all valves are closed and the ventricular myocardium contracts with closed valves (period of isometric contraction - Ic), so the pressure rises sharply in the ventricles (arrows point upwards): in the left ventricle to 70-80 mmHg, and in the right ventricle - to 12-15 mmHg. Ic lasts for 0.02-0.03s. In Fig.3, the flap valves are closed and the semilunar valves are open and the period of ejection (E) of ventricular systole begins, the arrows indicate the direction of blood flow: from the left ventricle blood flows into the aorta (the beginning of the great circle of circulation), and from the right ventricle - into the pulmonary artery (the beginning of the small circle of circulation). At the beginning of the expulsion period, the pressure in the ventricles continues to increase: in the left ventricle to 110-120 mmHg, and in the right ventricle - to 20-25 mmHg). E lasts for 0.28-0.32s. In Fig.4 the flap valves are closed and the semilunar valves are still open, the absence of the arrow shows that the expulsion of blood from the ventricles has stopped, as the pressure in the ventricles and the main vessels (aorta and pulmonary artery) is the same. This is the first period of diastole - protodiastolic (P) and this period lasts for 0.015-0.02 s. In Fig.5, the flap valves are closed and the semilunar valves are also closed due to the backflow of blood from the main vessels into the ventricles of the heart as the pressure in the ventricles decreases. The arrows indicate a sudden decrease in pressure in the ventricles of the heart to 0 - this period is called isometric relaxation (IR) - this period lasts for 0.08s. In Fig.6, the semilunar valves are closed and the flap valves are open. In contrast to Figure 1, in this case, the arrows indicate that blood from the atria flows into the ventricles, i.e. the ventricular filling period begins: passive filling occurs during atrial diastole (0.17s) and active filling occurs during atrial systole (0.1s). Thus, Figures 1,2,3 reflect different periods of the ventricular systole phase: 1 - AC; 2 - Ic; 3 - E. Figures 4,5,6 reflect different periods of the ventricular diastole phase: 4 - P; 5 - IR; 6 - ventricular filling period.

Figure 1 shows the synchronous recording of ECG (recording of myocardial excitation) and PCG (recording of heart sounds occurring during different phases of the cardiac cycle). There are 4 tones (I, II, III and IV) on the ECG: I tone occurs during ventricular systole, therefore called the systolic tone and consists of the following components: tension of the tendons of the leaflets

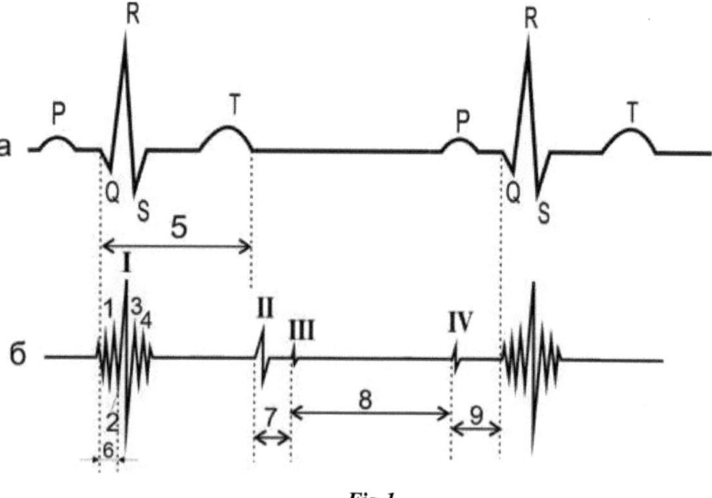

Fig.1

valves (1); closure of the flap valves - the beginning of high-amplitude oscillations (2); opening of the semilunar valves (3) and exit of the first portion of blood from the ventricles into the main vessels (4). Tone II occurs during diastole, when blood returning to the ventricles slams the semilunar valves, which is the cause of its occurrence, followed by isometric relaxation of the ventricles. III tone occurs during diastole, 0.08 s after the slamming of the semilunar valves and its cause is the opening of the flap valves and begins the period of filling of the ventricles of the heart. The IV tone occurs during diastole with active ventricular filling during atrial systole. I and II tones are always noted on the FCG, and III and IV tones in 10-15% of cases. Thus, four tones occur in one cardiac cycle: one during systole (I tone) and the others during diastole (II, III and IV tones). From this synchronous recording, the following periods of the cardiac cycle structure can be determined: duration of the cardiac cycle (RR interval on the ECG), duration of electrical systole (5-interval Q-T on the ECG), period of asynchronous ventricular systole contraction (6-interval from the beginning of the Q ECG to the beginning of the high-amplitude oscillation of the I tone on the FCG), duration of the period of isometric relaxation of the ventricular diastole phase (7-interval from II tone of ECG to III tone), duration of the period of passive filling of the ventricular diastole phase (8-interval from III tone of ECG to IV tone) and duration of active filling (9-interval from IV tone of ECG to the beginning of Q ECG).

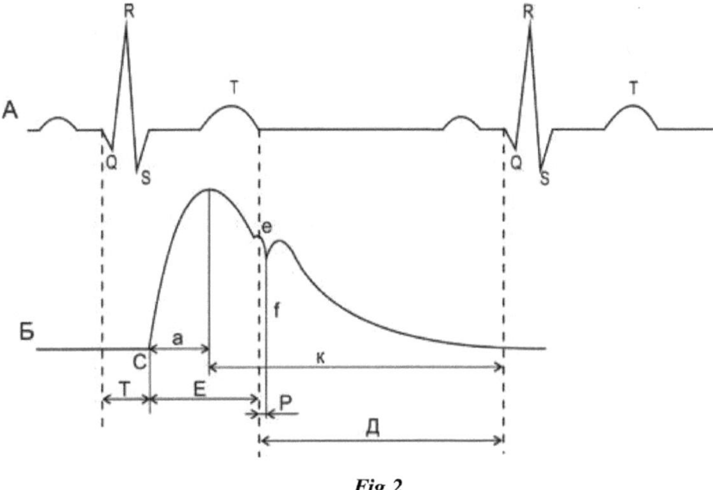

Fig.2

Fig.2 shows synchronous recording of ECG (A - recording of myocardial excitation biocurrents) and sphygmogram (B-SG - recording of arterial pulse). The SG distinguishes between the ascending part - anacrota (a) and the descending part - catacrota (k). Point e on the catacrota reflects the beginning of diastole (the beginning of the protodiastolic period - P), point f - slamming of the semilunar valves, the beginning of the dicrotic rise and the end of P. The following periods of the cardiac cycle structure can be identified on this synchronous recording: cardiac cycle duration (RR interval on ECG); duration of electrical systole (Q-T interval on ECG); tension phase (T - interval from the beginning of Q on ECG to point C on SG), which consists of periods of asynchronous and isometric contraction. This phase reflects the duration

47

of preparation of the heart for the useful work of expelling blood from the ventricles of the heart; the phase of expulsion of blood from the ventricles of the heart (E - the interval from the point C of the SG to the point e); the first period of diastole - the protodiastolic period (P - the interval from the point e of the SG to the point f); the duration of the entire diastole of the ventricles (D-interval from the point e of the SG to the beginning of Q ECG).

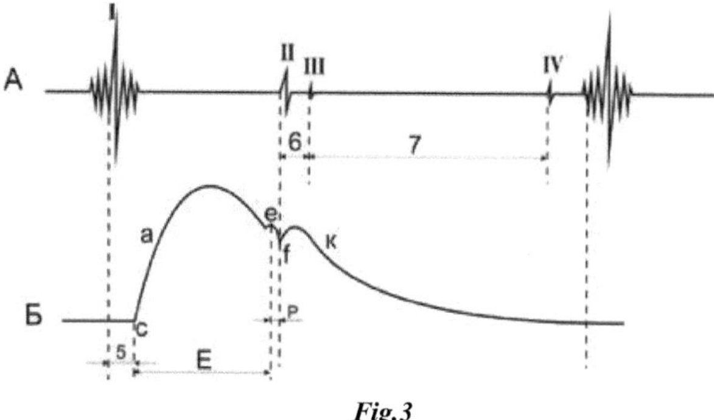

Fig.3

Fig.3 shows the synchronous recording of PPCG (A - recording of heart sounds occurring in different phases of the cardiac cycle) and sphygmogram (B-SG - recording of arterial pulse). There are 4 tones (I, II, III and IV) noted on the FCG: I tone occurs during ventricular systole, therefore called systolic tone and consists of the following components: tension of the tendons of the leaf valves (1); closure of the leaf valves - the beginning of high-amplitude oscillations (2); opening of the semilunar valves (3) and exit of the first portion of blood from the ventricles into the main vessels (4). II tone occurs during diastole, when blood returning to the ventricles slams the semilunar valves, which is the cause of its occurrence, followed by isometric relaxation of the ventricles. III tone occurs during diastole, 0.08 seconds after the slamming of semilunar valves and its cause is the opening of the leaf valves and begins the period of filling of the ventricles of the heart. The IV tone occurs during ventricular diastole with active ventricular filling during atrial systole. I and II tones are always noted on the FCG, and III and IV tones in 10-15% of cases. Thus, four tones occur during one cardiac cycle: one during systole (I tone), the others during diastole (II, III and IV tones). The SG distinguishes between the ascending part - anacrota (a) and the descending part - catacrota (k). Point e on the catacrota reflects the beginning of diastole (the beginning of the protodiastolic period - P), point f - slamming of the semilunar valves, the beginning of the dicrotic rise and the end of P. The following periods of the cardiac cycle structure can be identified on this synchronous recording: duration of the period of isometric contraction of ventricular systole (5-Ic - interval from the beginning of the high-amplitude oscillation of the I tone to the beginning of anacrta on SG point c); the phase of blood expulsion from the ventricles of the heart (E - interval from SG point c to point e); first period of diastole - protodiastolic period (P - interval from point e of SG to point f); duration of isometric relaxation period of ventricular diastole phase (6-interval from II tone of FCG to III tone); duration of

48

passive filling period of ventricular diastole phase (7-interval from III tone of FCG to IV tone).

Heart regulation

Figure 4 shows the sympathetic regulation of the heart. Three cervical ganglia (upper - 1, middle - 2 and lower - 3), as well as neurons in the lateral horns of the spinal cord of the upper five cervical ganglia are involved in sympathetic regulation of the heart.

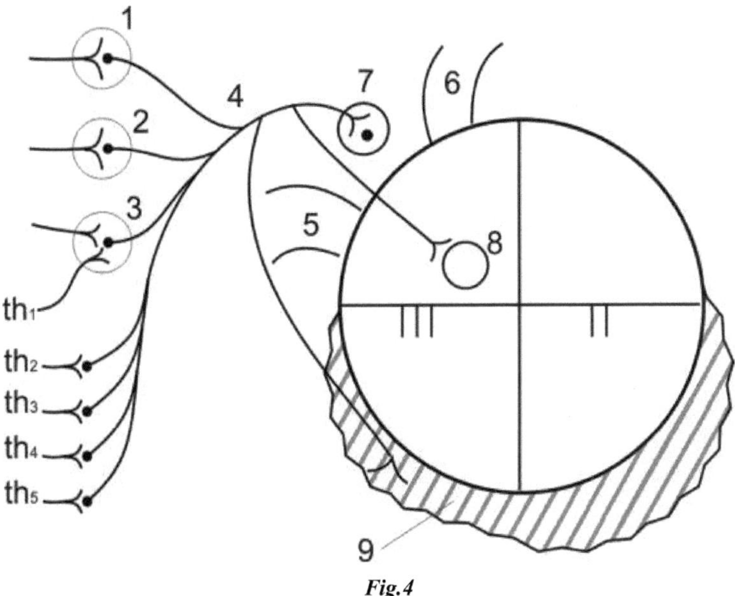

Fig.4

thoracic segments (th1-th5). The preganglionic fibres of th1 neurons terminate in the inferior cervical ganglion, forming the stellate ganglion. Postganglionic fibres of the sympathetic nerve from the cervical and paravertebral ganglia th2-th5 (4) terminate in the sinoatrial (CA-7) node, atrioventricular (AV-8) node and beta-1 adrenoreactive structures of the myocardium of the right and left ventricles (9). The nerve endings of the postganglionic fibre of the sympathetic nerve release noradrenaline. When noradrenaline interacts with P cells of the SA node, the rate of slow diastolic depolarisation increases, which leads to an increase in the number of impulses generated in the SA node and an increase in HR (tachycardia) - this is a positive chronotropic effect. When noradrenaline interacts with beta-1 adrenoreactive structures of ventricular myocardium, there is an increase in myocardial excitability (positive butmotropic effect), conduction (positive dromotropic effect) and contractility (positive inotropic effect).

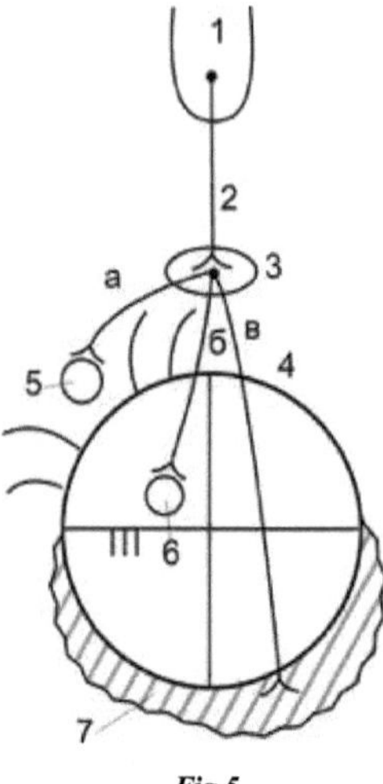

Fig.5 shows the parasympathetic regulation of heart function, in which the vagus nerve takes part, the nucleus of which is located in the medulla oblongata (1). The preganglionary fibre of the vagus nerve (2) ends in the intra-mural ganglion (3). Post-ganglionic fibres of the vagus nerve (a,b,c) respectively end in the sinoatrial node (SA - 5), atrioventricular node (AV - 6) and M-cholinoreactive structures of the myocardium of the right and left ventricles (7). Acetylcholine is released in the nerve endings of the postganglionic vagus nerve fibre. When acetylcholine interacts with P cells of the SA node, the rate of slow diastolic depolarisation decreases, which leads to a decrease in the number of impulses generated in the SA node and a decrease in HR (bradycardia) - this is a negative chronotropic effect. When acetylcholine interacts with M cholinoreactive structures of ventricular myocardium, there is a decrease in myocardial

Fig.5

excitability (negative butmotropic effect), conduction (negative dromotropic effect) and contractility (negative inotropic effect).

Fig.6 shows the intracardiac peripheral reflex that provides self-regulation of cardiac function. This reflex starts with excitation of myocardial stretch receptors (b) during ventricular diastole (ventricles are filled with blood, which leads to myocardial

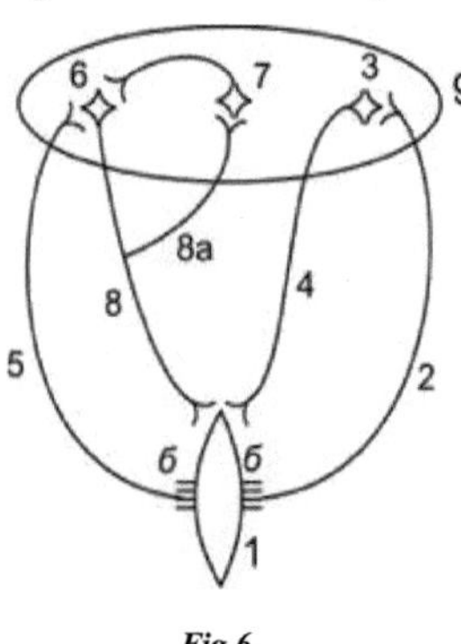

Fig.6

stretch). When these receptors are excited, impulses via afferent pathways (2 and 5) are simultaneously delivered to adrenergic (6) and cholinergic (3) neurons of the intramural ganglion (9). In this case, only the adrenergic neuron is excited (its excitability is greater than that of the cholinergic neuron) and in the nerve endings of the efferent fibre of the adrenergic neuron (8) norepinephrine is released, which interacts with beta-1 adrenoreactive structures of myocardium and there is an increase in myocardial excitability (positive butmotropic effect), conduction (positive dromotropic effect) and contractility (positive inotropic effect). At strong myocardial stretching there is an excitation of cholinergic neuron (3) and at the same time on collateral (8a) of efferent fibre of adrenergic neuron (8) impulses arrive to inhibitory neuron (7) excitation of which inhibits adrenergic neuron (6). Thus, under strong stretching, acetylcholine is released in the efferent fibre terminals of the cholinergic neuron (noradrenaline release in the efferent fibre terminals of the adrenergic neuron stops), which interacts with M-cholinoreactive structures of the myocardium, resulting in a decrease in myocardial excitability (negative batmotropic effect), conduction (negative dromotropic effect) and contractility (negative inotropic effect)

Figure 7 shows the change in cardiac performance when sympathetic and parasympathetic regulation is maintained (a) and after the

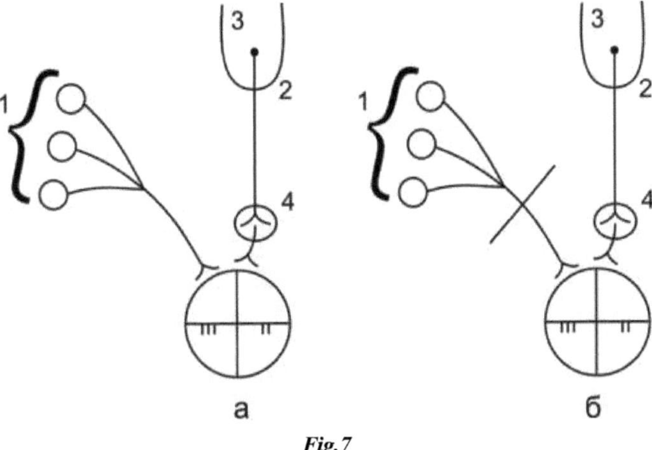

Fig.7

transection of the sympathetic nerve (b): 1 - cervical ganglia, where postganglionic fibres of the sympathetic nerve begin; 2 - medulla oblongata; 3 - nucleus of the vagus nerve, which performs parasympathetic regulation of the heart; 4 - intramural ganglion, where the preganglionic fibre of the vagus nerve ends and the postganglionic fibre begins. As a result of this experiment it is noted that HR after transection of the sympathetic nerve practically does not change. This result indicates that the sympathetic nerve centre of the heart has no tone, i.e. in the resting state the heart does not receive impulses along the fibres of the sympathetic nerve.

Fig.8 shows the change of heart work with preservation of sympathetic and parasympathetic regulation (a) and after cutting of parasympathetic nerve (b): 1 - cervical ganglia where postganglionic fibres of sympathetic nerve start; 2 - medulla oblongata; 3 - nucleus of vagus nerve, which carries out parasympathetic regulation of heart work; 4 - intramural ganglion, where preganglionic fibres of sympathetic nerve end.

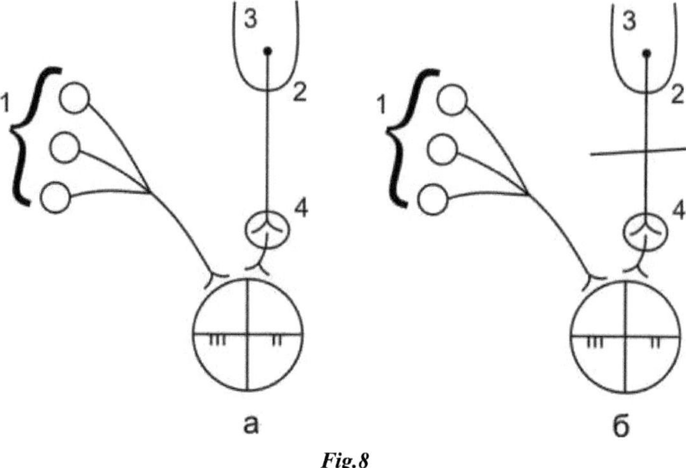

Fig.8

fibre of the vagus nerve and the postganglionic fibre begins. As a result of this experiment, it is noted that after transection of the parasympathetic nerve, HR increases sharply (from 70-80 beats/min to 130-140 beats/min). This result indicates that the nucleus of the vagus nerve has tone, that is, it is in constant excitation. Thus, at rest, the heart is constantly under the influence of the vagus nerve.

Fig.9 shows the change of heart work with preservation of sympathetic and parasympathetic regulation (a) and after transection of sympathetic and parasympathetic nerves (b): 1 - cervical ganglia from where postganglionary fibres of sympathetic nerve begin; 2 - medulla oblongata; 3 - nucleus of vagus nerve, carrying out parasympathetic regulation of heart work; 4 - intramural ganglion, where preganglionary fibre of vagus nerve ends and postganglionary fibre begins. As a result of this experiment it is noted that after simultaneous transection of sympathetic and parasympathetic nerves sharply increased

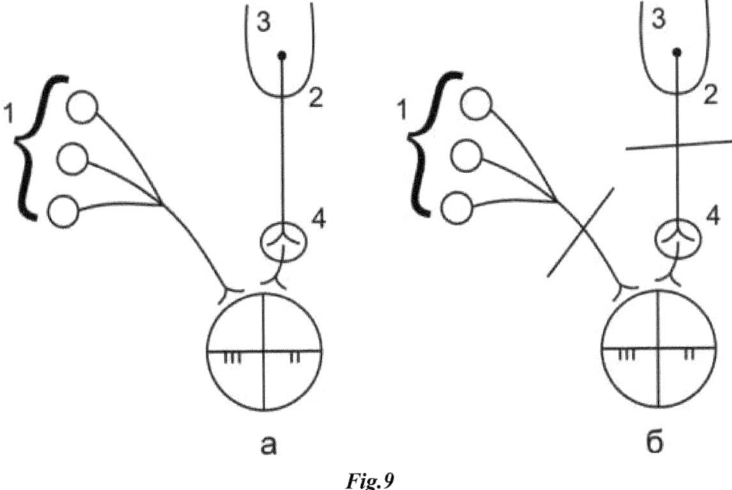

a   б

Fig.9

HR (from 70-80 beats/min to 130-140 beats/min). This result indicates that the resting heart receives impulses only from the vagus nerve, i.e. the resting heart is constantly under the influence of the vagus nerve and does not receive impulses from the sympathetic nerve.

Basic laws of haemodynamics. Systemic circulation. Blood pressure

Figure 10 shows the movement of blood from the heart (A), through the arterial part of the vascular system (B), through the capillaries (C) and the venous part of the vascular system. The movement of blood from the heart is pulsatile and intermittent: during systole (1) blood comes out of the ventricles and during diastole (2) there is no blood. In the arterial part of the vascular system, blood movement is pulsatile and continuous. The continuity of blood flow in the arterial part is due to the aortic compression chamber, which is formed during ventricular systole due to the

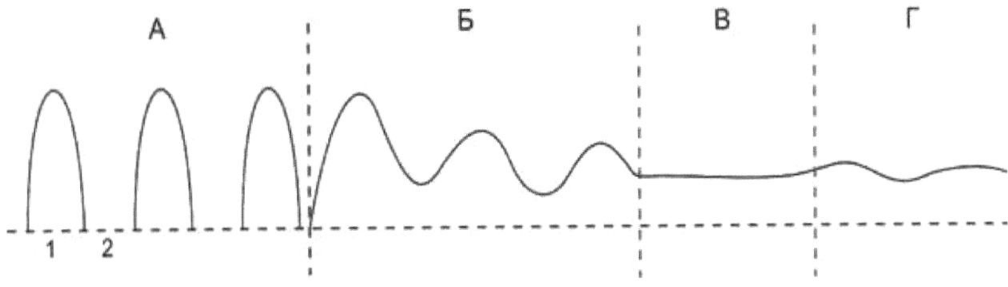

Fig.10

the presence of a large number of elastic fibres in the middle layer of the aorta. This chamber is filled with blood during ventricular systole, which exits during ventricular diastole. In the capillary part, blood movement is non-pulsatile and continuous, while in the venous part of the vascular system, blood movement is weakly pulsatile (due to periodic congestion occurring during one cardiac cycle) and continuous.

Figure 11 shows the relationship between pressure (P) in different part of the vascular system (1-aorta, 2-large calibre arteries, 3-medium calibre arteries, 4-arterioles, 5-capillaries, 6-venules, 7-venules, 8-hollow veins) and resistance(R). As can be seen

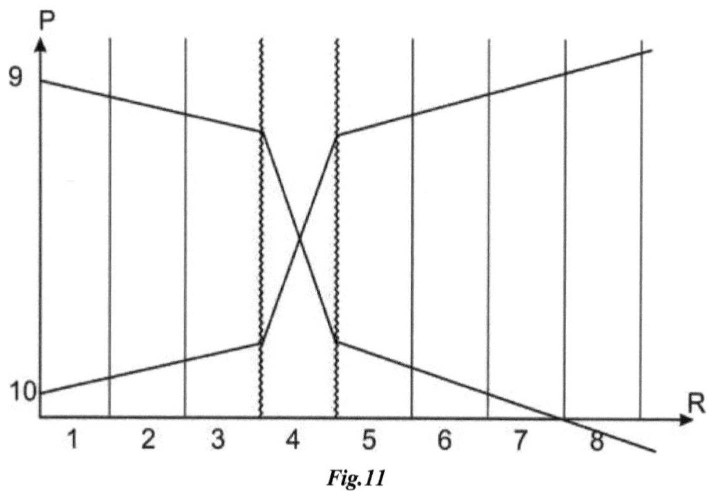

Fig.11

from the figure, this dependence is inversely proportional: the smaller the resistance (10), the greater the pressure (9) in the vessel. In each subsequent vessel, the resistance is composed of the resistance of this vessel and the sum of the resistances of the previous vessels. The smallest resistance is in the aorta, as this vessel is closest to the heart (pump) - here the highest pressure (100 mmHg). The greatest resistance is in the vena cava - the vessel furthest from the heart (pump), so it has the lowest pressure (-5 mmHg). Part of the heart's energy is spent to pressurise the vessel wall and part of it is spent to overcome resistance: the closer the vessel is to the heart (aorta), the more energy is spent on pressure and less on overcoming resistance; the further the vessel is from the heart (hollow veins), the less energy is left for pressure and more is spent on overcoming resistance. The figure shows that the greatest pressure drop (the difference between the pressure at the beginning of the vessel and at the end) is in the arterioles (4). This is due to the fact that the middle layer of arterioles has the largest number of smooth muscle cells and arterioles cause the greatest resistance to blood flow.

Figure 12 shows the relationship between the linear velocity of blood through vessels (V) in different parts of the vascular system (1 - aorta, 2 - large-calibre arteries, 3 - medium-calibre arteries, 4 - arterioles, 5 - capillaries, 6 - venules, 7 - veins, 8 -

hollow veins) and the total cross-section of the vessel (S). As can be seen from the figure, this dependence is inversely proportional: the smaller the total cross-section (10), the greater the linear velocity (9) in the vessel. The smallest cross-section is in the aorta (1), so the linear velocity is the highest here and is 0.5 m/sec. The largest total cross-section in the capillaries (5 - 400-600 times larger than in the aorta), so here is the smallest linear velocity and is 0.001 m/sec. The total cross-section of the two hollow veins is twice as large as that of the aorta, so the linear velocity in the hollow veins is approximately twice as small and is about 0.25 m/sec.

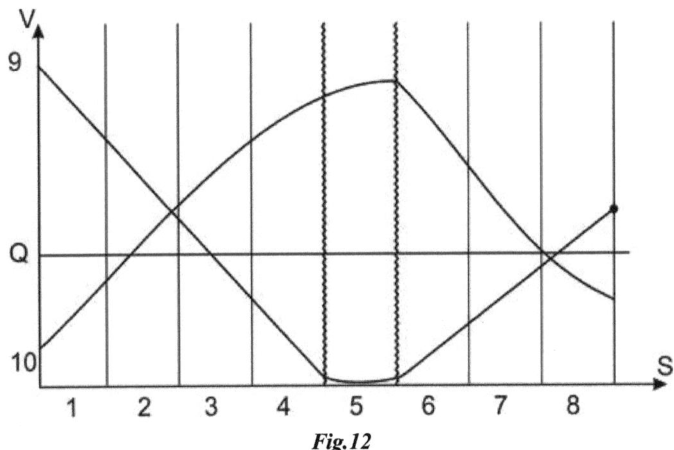

Fig.12

Volumetric velocity (Q-quantity of blood passed through the cross-section of a vessel per unit time) is the same in all vessels, as this velocity depends on HR and systolic blood volume (Q = HR x juice), i.e. on the work of the heart. If 5 litres of blood leave the ventricles of the heart per minute, then 5 litres of blood passes through the total cross-section of each vessel in one min.

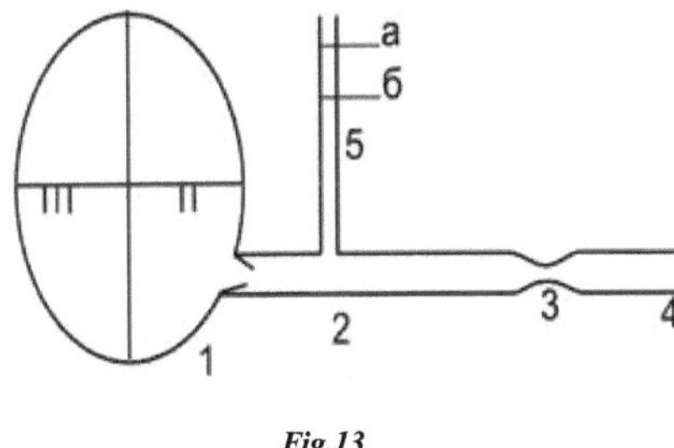

Fig.13

Fig.13 shows a model of the vascular system, from which we can see that two factors influence the value of BP (5) - the pressure on the wall of the entire arterial part of the vascular system from the aorta to the arterioles (2): volume velocity (Q) and resistance (R). Q depends on the work of the heart (Q=HSSxSOC): the greater Q, the greater BP (a); as Q decreases, BP also decreases (b). R depends on the state of smooth muscle cells (SMCs) of arterioles (3): when SMCs contract, arterioles narrow, resistance increases and BP increases (a), when SMCs relax, arterioles dilate, resistance decreases and BP decreases (b). Thus, it follows from this model that BP depends on two factors, which can be expressed by the following formula: BP = QxR, i.e. BP is directly proportional to volume velocity and resistance: the greater Q and R, the greater BP.

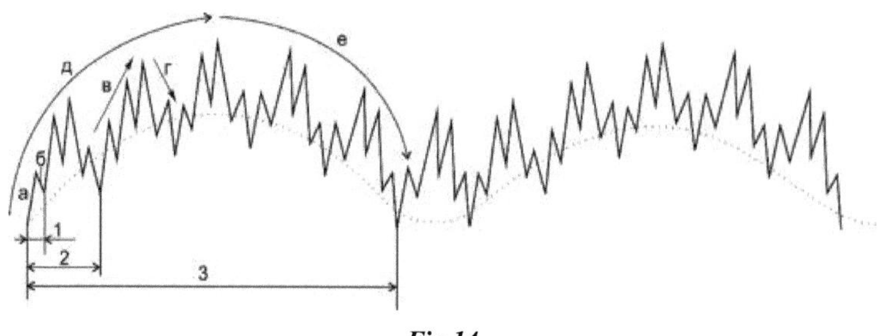

Fig.14

Fig.14 shows the BP curve, which shows waves of three orders, differing in period. Wave of order I (1), the period of which corresponds to the duration of one cardiac cycle: during ventricular systole BP increases (a), during diastole BP decreases (b). II (2) order wave whose period corresponds to the duration of one respiratory cycle: during exhalation BP increases (c), during inhalation BP decreases (d). Wave III (3), the period of which corresponds to a change in the tone of the pressor section (P) of the vasomotor centre (VDC): when the tone of the VDC increases, the BP increases (e) due to vasoconstriction and increase in resistance (R); when the tone of the VDC decreases (when the depressor section of the VDC is excited), the BP decreases (f) due to vasoconstriction and decrease in R.

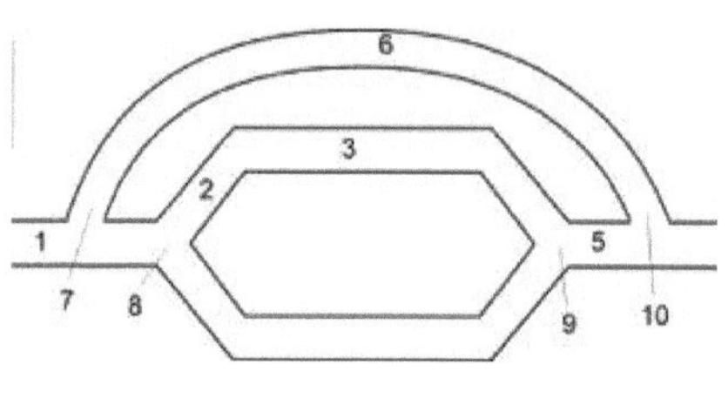

Fig.15

Fig.15 shows the microcirculatory bed, which consists of 6 vessels: 1. - Arterioles, the middle layer of which consists of a large number of smooth muscle cells (SMC). Arterioles participate in BP regulation by changing resistance: when SMCs contract, the vessel narrows, resistance increases and BP increases; when SMCs relax, the vessel expands, resistance decreases and BP decreases. Arterioles are also involved in the regulation of blood flow in capillaries, so this vessel I.M. Sechenov called the taps of the vascular system - when narrowing arterioles less blood enters capillaries, and when expanding - more. 2 - precapillary sphincters directly regulate the volume of incoming blood into the capillaries: when the GMC of precapillary sphincters contract, the blood filling of the capillary decreases, and when relaxed, the blood filling of the capillary increases. 3 - capillaries, or metabolic vessels, because here there is an exchange of water, substances and gases between the blood and tissues. 4 - postcapillary sphincters regulate the blood pressure in capillaries: when the GMCs of postcapillary sphincters contract, the intracapillary pressure increases, which contributes to transcapillary filtration (increases the transfer of fluid from blood to tissue), when the GMCs relax, the intracapillary pressure decreases and filtration decreases. 5 - venules, or collecting vessels, collect blood from capillaries. 6 - arterio-venous anastamoses, or shunting vessels, are involved in thermoregulation: at low ambient temperature the SMCs of precapillary sphincters reflexively contract and blood bypassing the capillary bed passes through the shunting vessels, reducing heat dissipation; at increasing ambient temperature the SMCs of precapillary sphincters reflexively relax and blood passes through the capillary bed, thus increasing heat dissipation. The gas composition of blood taken in areas 7, 8, 10 does not differ, because in area 7, 8 there was no gas exchange yet, and in area 10 blood passed through the bypass vessel, where there is no gas exchange. The blood in region 9 differs from blood 7,8,10 in that there is less oxygen and more carbon dioxide, as this blood has passed through capillaries where gas exchange takes place (O2 enters the tissue and CO2 enters the blood from the tissue).

Circulatory regulation

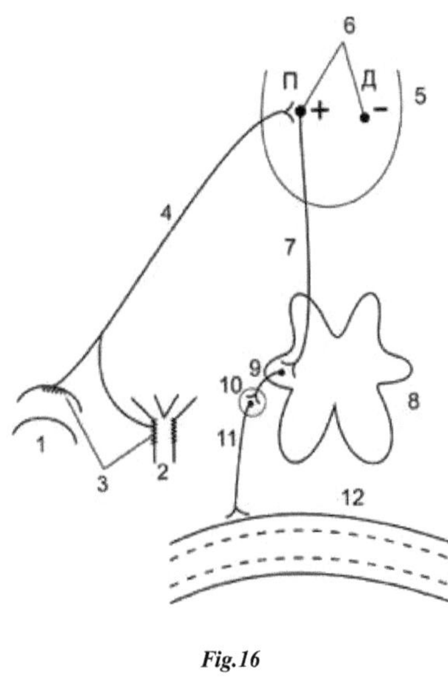

Fig.16

Figure 16 shows the pressor reflex, which is accompanied by an increase in BP. Receptors of this reflex are located in the aortic arch (1) and in the place of bifurcation of the common carotid artery into external and internal (2) and are called chemoreceptors (3 - CR). An adequate stimulus of CP is a decrease of oxygen tension in arterial blood (RO2). The threshold value of RO2, at which CPs are excited, corresponds to 160-180 mm Hg, and the maximum oxygen tension in arterial blood under normal conditions (0 m above sea level at atmospheric pressure of 760 mm Hg) can be 100 mm Hg. It follows that in the state of rest the CP are in constant excitation and from the CP constantly impulses go along afferent pathways (4) to the pressor section (P) of the vasomotor centre (VDC-6), which is located in the medulla oblongata (5). Upon excitation of P, there is a reciprocal inhibition of the depressor section of the SDC (D) and through efferent pathways (7) impulses arrive in the lateral horns of the spinal cord of the thoracic and lumbar segments (8). From here the preganglionic fibre (9) of the sympathetic nerve (vasoconstrictor) to the sympathetic ganglion (10) begins, from here the postganglionic fibre (11) begins and terminates in the vascular SMC (12). The endings of the postganglionic fibre release norepinephrine, which interacts with alpha or beta1 adrenergic structures of the SMCs, causing their contraction, vasoconstriction, vasoconstriction, increased resistance and BP rise.

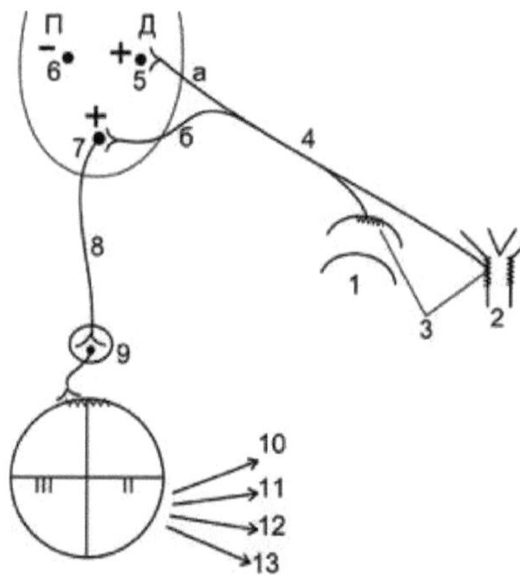

Fig.17

Figure 17 shows the depressor reflex, which is accompanied by a decrease in BP. Receptors of this reflex are located in the aortic arch (1) and at the bifurcation of the common carotid artery into external and internal (2) and are called baroreceptors (3 - BR). An adequate stimulus for BP is an increase in BP. When BP increases, BP excitation occurs. Impulses from the BR through the afferent pathway (4a) reach the depressor section (D) of the vasomotor centre (VDC). Excitation of the D leads to a reciprocal inhibition of the pressor section (P) of the VDC, the tone of P decreases, which leads to vascular dilation, decreased resistance, and BP decreases. In addition, impulses from the BR via afferent pathways (4b) reach the nucleus of the vagus nerve and increase its tone (excitation). Impulses along preganglionary fibres of the vagus nerve (8) reach the intramural ganglion (9) and along postganglionary fibres (8a) reach the sinoatrial node (SA) and ventricular myocardium. Acetyl-choline is released at the endings of postganglionary fibres, which interacts with P cells of the SA node (decreases HR - bradycardia - negative chronotropic effect - 10) and M-choline-reactive structures of the ventricular myocardium (decreases myocardial excitability - negative butmotropic effect - 11, myocardial conduction decreases - negative dromotropic effect - 12, myocardial contraction force decreases - negative inotropic effect - 13). Thus, during the depressor reflex, BP reduction occurs due to a decrease in volume velocity (vagus nucleus tone increases) and resistance (excitation of D SDC causing reciprocal inhibition of P SDC).

BLOOD PHYSIOLOGY

Blood and its properties

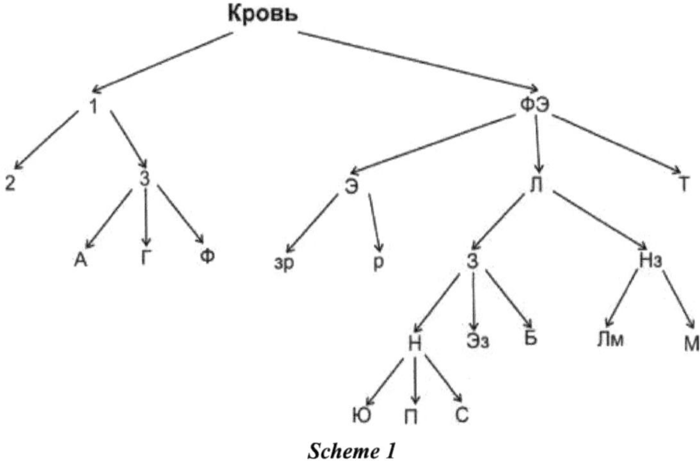

Scheme 1

Scheme 1 shows the components of blood: 1) plasma; 2) inorganic substances; 3) organic substances (proteins: A - albumin, G - globulin, F - fibrinogen); 4) blood formed elements (BFE): E - erythrocytes (r - mature, p - young erythrocytes, reticulocytes); L - leucocytes: Z - granular (N - neutrophils: y - young, p - bacillary, s - segmented; Ez - eosinophils; B - basophils); Nz - non-grained (Lm - lymphocytes, M - monocytes); T - platelets.

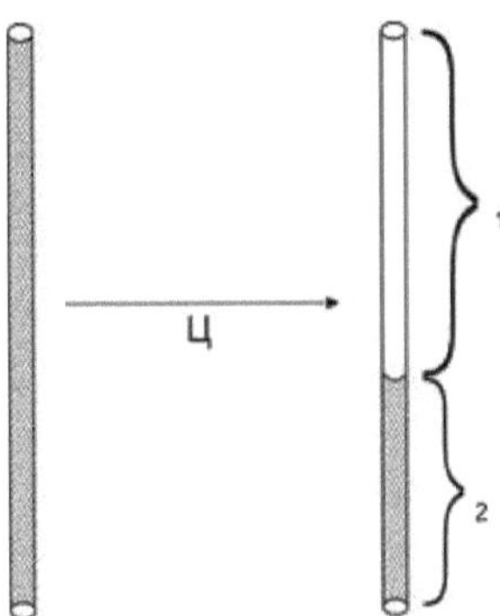

Fig.18

Figure 18 shows how to determine the haematocrit, or haematocrit (percentage of the blood's form elements):

A-capillary with blood before centrifugation; B-capillary with blood after centrifugation (blood divided into two components: 1-Plasma (the majority and normal is 55%-60%), 2-Formen elements (the smaller part and normal is 40%-45%).

Figure 19 shows a test tube with 0.5% sodium chloride solution (hypotonic solution). Erythrocytes with different osmotic resistance (osmotic resistance of erythrocyte is the highest concentration of hypotonic solution at which the destruction of erythrocyte shell occurs) are placed in this test tube - the value of its osmotic resistance is marked inside the erythrocytes. The figure shows that the greatest resistance to hypotonic solution has erythrocyte with resistance 0.38% (the shell of this erythrocyte is destroyed in 0.38% solution, and in 0.5% this erythrocyte swells) and the least resistance to hypotonic solution has erythrocyte with resistance 0.6%, as the shell of this erythrocyte is destroyed in 0.6% solution, and in 0.5% solution more water penetrates into this

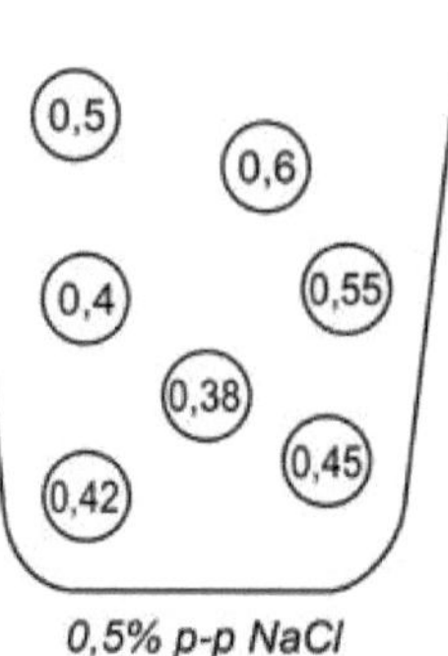

0,5% p-p NaCl

Fig.19

erythrocyte than in 0.6% (the less concentration of hypotonic solution, the more water from the solution penetrates into the erythrocyte), so the shell of this erythrocyte is destroyed in this solution. Thus, all erythrocytes with an osmotic resistance of 0.5% or more (0.6%; 0.55% and 0.5%) are in this solution. Erythrocytes whose osmotic resistance is less than 0.5% (0.45%; 0.42%; 0.4% and 0.38%) swell. Since erythrocytes have different osmotic resistance but the same osmotic pressure (in normal conditions, the osmotic pressure of an erythrocyte corresponds to the osmotic pressure of 0.9% sodium chloride solution), therefore all erythrocytes whose resistance is less than 0.5% swell equally.

	норм	Ацидоз		Алкалоз	
		комп.	некомп.	комп.	некомп.
pH	m	m_1	m_2	m_3	m_4
БЕк	n	n_1	n_2	n_3	n_4
БЕщ	p	p_1	p_2	p_3	p_4

The acid-base equilibrium of the blood can be determined using the hydrogen balance (pH) and buffer capacity (BC). In normal blood pH ranges from 7.36 to 7.42 units, i.e. blood is normally slightly alkaline. A decrease in pH is noted when the blood is acidified (acidosis), and an increase in pH when the blood is alkalised (alkalosis). The BE of blood is determined by the amount of acid (buffer capacity for acid - BEc) or alkali (buffer capacity for alkali - BEh) that must be added to 1 litre of buffer solution (blood) to change the pH of this solution by 1 unit. For example, 2 litres of alkali was added to 1 litre of blood with pH=7.36, after which the pH of the blood became 8.36 (pH increased by 1 unit), hence the BEC of this blood is 2 litres. If 31 of acid was added to 1l of blood with pH=7.36, after which the pH of the blood became 6.36 (pH decreased by 1 unit), hence the BEc of this blood is 3l. According to the change of pH or BE, there is a distinction between compensated (blood pH does not change, only Beck and BEC) acidosis and alkalosis and uncompensated (in this case changes in BEC and BEC are accompanied by changes in pH). In this table it is necessary to show how pH, Beck and BECh of normal blood differs from blood with compensated and uncompensated acidosis and alkalosis: m=m1=m3; m>m2; m<m4; m2<m4. n>n1>n2; n<n3<n4. p<p1<p2; p>p3>p4.

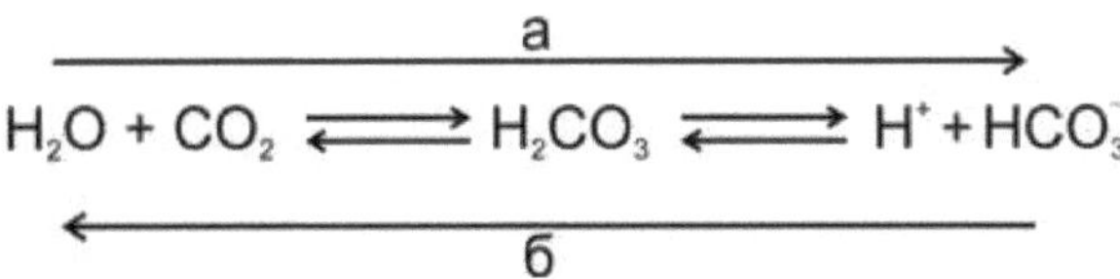

This diagram shows the mechanism of blood pH regulation due to changes in lung function: a) decrease in lung function (hypoventilation), in this case CO2 accumulates in the blood, carbonic acid is formed, which dissociates into hydrogen cation and anion HCO3, which leads to an increase in hydrogen ions and blood pH decreases. Prolonged hypoventilation can lead to acidosis; b) increase in lung function (hyperventilation), this results in an intense release of CO2 from the blood, which leads to a decrease in hydrogen ions in the blood and an increase in blood pH. Prolonged hyperventilation leads to alkalosis.

Fig.19 shows the role of oncotic pressure (P - part of osmotic pressure due to plasma proteins, normal is 25-30 mmHg) in regulation of water exchange between blood (1) and tissues (2). The magnitude of the arrow shows the amount of water permeating into the tissue at normal P (a), when P increases above normal (b), and when P decreases below normal (c). A sharp increase in oncotic pressure (b) is observed when the amount of plasma proteins increases. In this case, due to hydrophilicity of proteins (like water), water is retained in the vascular bed. This leads, on the one hand, to skin dryness,

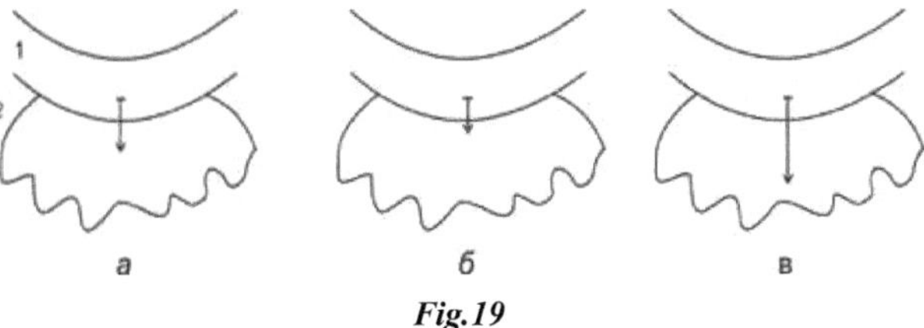

Fig.19

and, on the other hand, to increase the volume of circulating blood at the expense of the liquid part (plasma), which leads to a decrease in haematocrit and an increase in BP (due to an increase in volumetric velocity). A sharp decrease in oncotic pressure (c) is noted with a decrease in the amount of plasma proteins. In this case, water is not retained in the vascular bed and freely penetrates into the tissue. This leads, on the one hand, to tissue oedema (starvation or protein-free oedema), and on the other hand, to a decrease in the volume of circulating blood at the expense of the liquid part (plasma), which leads to an increase in haematocrit and a decrease in BP (due to a decrease in volume velocity).

Blood Form Elements.
Haemoglobin, its types and compounds

Diagram 2 shows the constituent parts of the blood formational elements (FE): E - erythrocytes (h - mature, p - young erythrocytes, reticulocytes); T - platelets; L - leucocytes: H - granular (N - neutrophils: y - young, p - bacillary, s - segmented; Ez - eosinophils; B - basophils); Nz - non-grained (Lm - lymphocytes, M - monocytes).

Fig.20 shows the change in the percentage of neutrophils and lymphocytes (N/L) during ontogeny (as a function of age -B). Of the whole leukaemia (percentage of

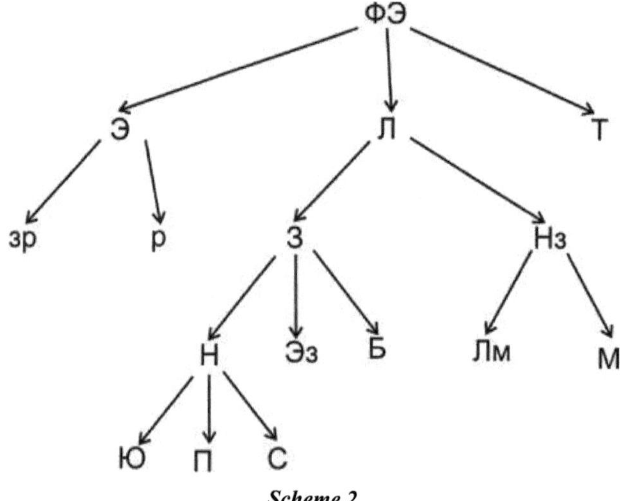

Scheme 2

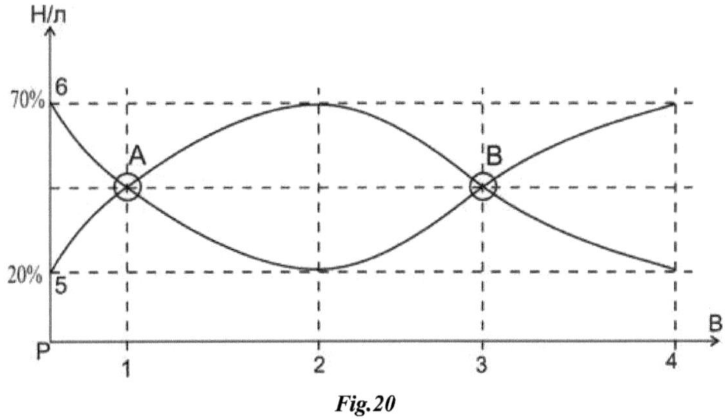

Fig.20

The percentage of neutrophils and lymphocytes only changes in ontogenesis: at birth (P) the percentage of neutrophils (70%) and lymphocytes (20%) corresponds to adult values. Further, the neutrophil content decreases and the lymphocyte content increases. By day 5-6 after birth (1), the number of neutrophils and lymphocytes becomes equal (first crossing - A). After the 6th day after birth, the number of neutrophils continues to decrease and the number of lymphocytes continues to increase and by 5-6 months after birth (2) the number of neutrophils becomes minimal and the number of lymphocytes becomes maximal. Then the number of lymphocytes decreases and the number of neutrophils increases and by 5-6 years of age (3) there is a second crossover (B), when the number of neutrophils corresponds to the number of lymphocytes. After the second crossover, neutrophil counts continue to increase and lymphocyte counts continue to decrease and by 14-16 years of age (4) are at adult levels (at birth).

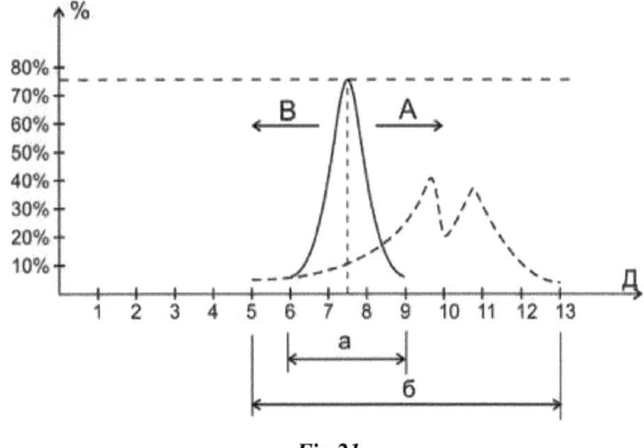

Fig.21

Figure 21 shows the anisocytosis curve showing the percentage (%) of different erythrocyte diameters (D). Each erythrocyte lives for about 3 months, so in peripheral blood there are erythrocytes of different ages that differ in their diameter. The diameter of erythrocytes in norm varies (differs) within 2.5-3 μ (difference between the maximum and minimum diameter of erythrocytes), the highest percentage of erythrocytes (75%) with a diameter of 7.2-7.5 μ.- this is the normal curve of anisocytosis (a). In anaemia (reduction in the number of red blood cells and haemoglobin), the anisocytosis curve may shift to the left (B) or right (A). The figure shows a rightward shift of the anisocytosis curve (b), which is seen in vitamin B12 deficiency anaemia. The curve shows that when the anisocytosis curve is shifted to the right, there is a dramatic increase in the variation of erythrocyte diameters within 7-8 μ - this strong variation in erythrocyte diameters is called poikilocytosis. When the anisocytosis curve is shifted to the right, the percentage of erythrocytes with a larger diameter increases, so the saturation of one erythrocyte with haemoglobin increases and there is an increase in the colour index (the degree of saturation of the erythrocyte with haemoglobin) greater than one (hyperchromic anaemia).

Blood clotting. Blood groups. Rhesus factor

Figure 22 shows the conditions under which the agglutination reaction (sticking of red blood cells together) occurs. Two conditions are necessary for the agglutination reaction: 1) the meeting of agglutinogens and agglutinins of the same name (agglutinogen A with agglutinin alpha; agglutinogen B with agglutinin beta); 2) a threshold concentration of agglutinins, since they, unlike agglutinogens, are capable of dilution in the recipient's plasma. The threshold concentration of agglutinins at which the agglutination reaction occurs corresponds to that observed at a dilution of 1:13. Thus, if the agglutinins are diluted more than 13-fold (1:14, 1:15, 1:16, etc.) in the recipient's blood they are

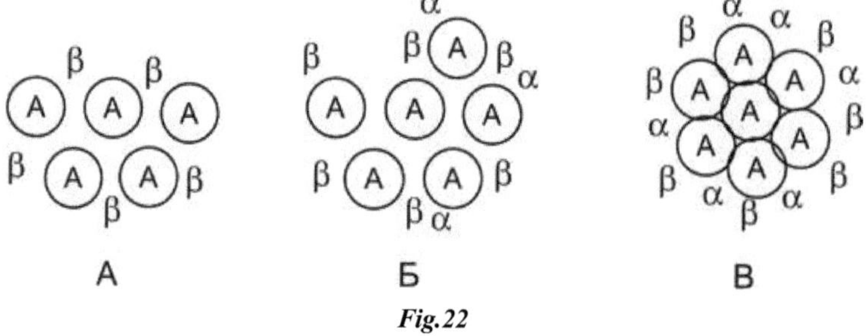

Fig.22

are not able to glue erythrocytes with the same agglutinogen, if the agglutinins are diluted in the recipient's blood by 13 times or less (1:13, 1:12, 1:11, etc.) they are able to glue erythrocytes with the same agglutinogen. Figure A shows the second blood group (agglutinogen A and agglutinin beta). Here, the above conditions are not met, so there is no agglutination reaction. In Figure B, a patient with group two has been supplemented with group three plasma, which contains alpha agglutinin. In this case, the first condition is met, but the second condition is not met - not enough plasma was added, so the alpha agglutinins are highly diluted (dilution of 1:14 or more), in this case there is no erythrocyte agglutination reaction. Figure B shows that the patient from the second group was added a large amount of plasma of the third group, so the concentration of agglutinins corresponds to a dilution of 1:13 or less, that is, in this case both conditions are met, so there is an agglutination reaction (all erythrocytes containing agglutinogen A adhered to each other due to the high concentration of alpha agglutinins).

Fig.23 shows the method of blood group determination using anti-A coliclone (which allows to determine the presence or absence of agglutinogen A in the erythrocytes of the tested blood), anti-B coliclone (which allows to determine the presence or absence of agglutinogen B in the erythrocytes of the tested blood) and anti-B coliclone (which allows to determine the presence or absence of agglutinogen B in the erythrocytes of the tested blood).

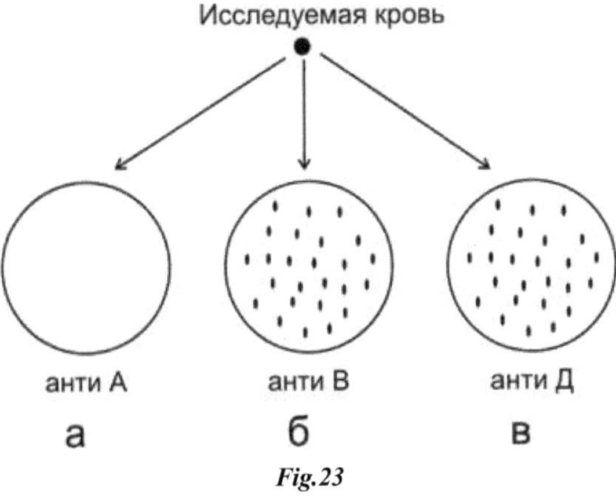

Fig.23

The anti-D ciliclone makes it possible to determine the presence (Rh positive blood) or absence (Rh negative blood) of agglutinogen D (Rh agglutinogen) in the erythrocytes of the tested blood. In this figure, after adding the blood under study to the wells with ciliclone anti A (a), anti B (b) and D (c), the agglutination reaction of the erythrocytes of the blood under study with ciliclone anti B and anti D occurred. The results show that the erythrocytes of the blood under study contain agglutinogen B (blood group III) and agglutinogen D (rhesus positive blood). Thus, the tested blood is blood group III (erythrocytes contain agglutinogen B and plasma contains agglutinin alpha) and Rhesus positive (erythrocytes contain Rhesus agglutinogen D in addition to agglutinogen B). The formula of the tested blood is III (Bα) Rh$^+$.

Fig.24 shows the method of blood group determination using anti-A coliclone (which allows to determine the presence or absence of agglutinogen A in the erythrocytes of the blood under study), anti-B coliclone (which allows to determine the presence or absence of agglutinogen B in the erythrocytes of the blood under study) and anti-B coliclone (which allows to determine the presence or absence of agglutinogen B in the erythrocytes of the blood under study).

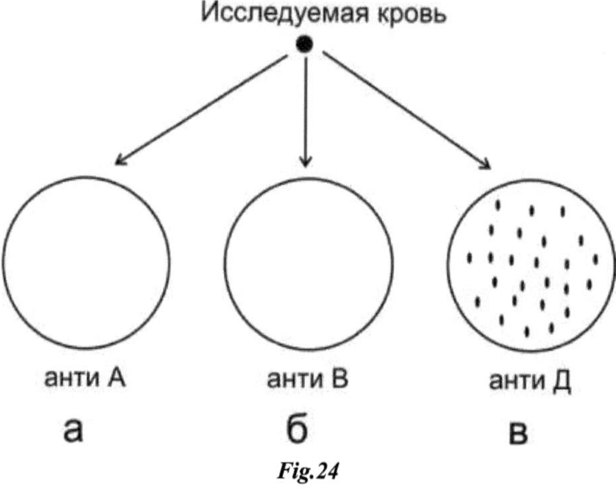

Fig.24

The anti-D cyclone makes it possible to determine the presence (rhesus positive blood) or absence (rhesus negative blood) of agglutinogen D (rhesus agglutinogen) in the erythrocytes of the tested blood. In this figure, after adding the test blood to the wells with anti-A (a), anti-B (b) and anti-D (c), the ag-glutination reaction of the test blood erythrocytes with anti-D agglutinogen occurred.

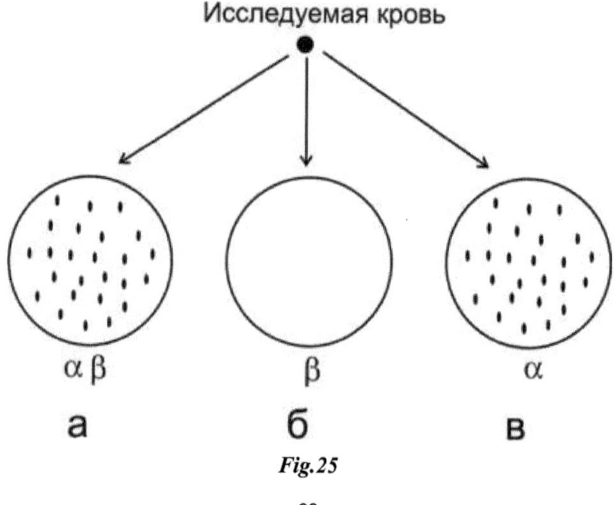

Fig.25

The results show that the erythrocytes of the tested blood do not contain agglutinogen A and B, but have agglutinogen D (Rhesus positive blood). Thus, the tested blood is group I (erythrocytes do not contain agglutinogens and plasma contains alpha and beta agglutinins) and Rh positive (erythrocytes contain only Rh agglutinogen D). The formula of the tested blood is I ($0\alpha\beta$) Rh^+.

Figure 25 shows the method of blood group determination using standard sera (serum is plasma without fibrinogen) of group I with alpha and beta agglutinins (a), group II with beta agglutinins and group III with alpha agglutinins. In this figure, after adding the test blood to the wells with alpha and beta agglutinins (a), beta (b) and alpha (c), the agglutination reaction of erythrocytes of the test blood in serum with alpha and beta agglutinins (a) and in serum with alpha agglutinins (c) occurred. The results indicate that the agglutination reaction occurred in those sera with agglutinin alpha (a and c), therefore, in the erythrocytes of the blood under study there was agglutinogen A, which corresponds to group II. Thus, the tested blood is of group II (in erythrocytes of which there is agglutinogen A and in plasma there is agglutinin beta). The formula of the tested blood is II ($A\beta$).

Figure 26 shows the method of blood group determination using standard sera (serum is plasma without fibrinogen) of group I with alpha and beta agglutinins (a), group II with beta agglutinins and group III with alpha agglutinins. In this figure, after adding the test blood to the wells with alpha and beta agglutinins (a), beta (b) and alpha (c), the agglutination reaction of the test blood erythrocytes occurred only in the serum with beta agglutinin (b). The results are doubtful, i.e. in this

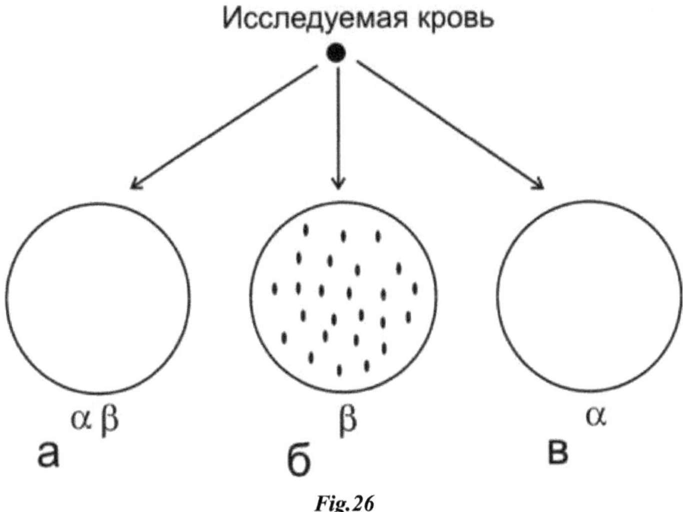

Fig.26

In this case the blood type cannot be determined. If an agglutination reaction has occurred in group II serum (there are beta agglutinins), then this reaction must also occur in group I serum (there are also beta agglutinins). Group I serum (a) serves as a control: if the agglutination reaction occurred in group II serum (b) or group III serum (c), it must necessarily occur in group I serum, where there are alpha and beta agglutinins. Thus, blood group cannot be determined from this result. It is necessary to repeat the result.

It is noted in Fig.27 that when group I blood (a - donor) is added to a recipient with group II blood (b), there may be an agglutination reaction of the recipient's erythrocytes (1), or there may be no agglutination reaction (2). This depends on the amount of group I blood that is added to the recipient with group II blood. When group I blood is added to a recipient with group II blood, the danger is agglutinins alpha in the donor's blood, which may promote agglutination of the recipient's erythrocytes having agglutinogen A (meeting of agglutinogens and agglutinins of the same name: agglutinogen A meets agglutinin alpha). In this case, the agglutination reaction depends on a sufficient concentration of agglutinins, as they, unlike agglutinogens, can be diluted in the recipient's plasma. The threshold concentration of agglutinins at which the agglutination reaction occurs corresponds to that observed at a dilution of 1:13. In the first case (b1), a large amount of group I blood was added and the concentration of alpha agglutinins in the recipient's plasma corresponds to a dilution of 1:13 or less (1:12; 1:11, etc.). In the second case (b2), a small amount of blood was added and the concentration of donor blood alpha agglutinins in the recipient's plasma corresponds to a dilution of 1:14 or more (1:15, 1:16, etc.), so there is no agglutination reaction here, although the condition of the meeting of agglutinogens and agglutinins of the same name is met (the meeting of the recipient's agglutinogen A meets the donor's alpha agglutinin, which is diluted in the recipient's plasma).

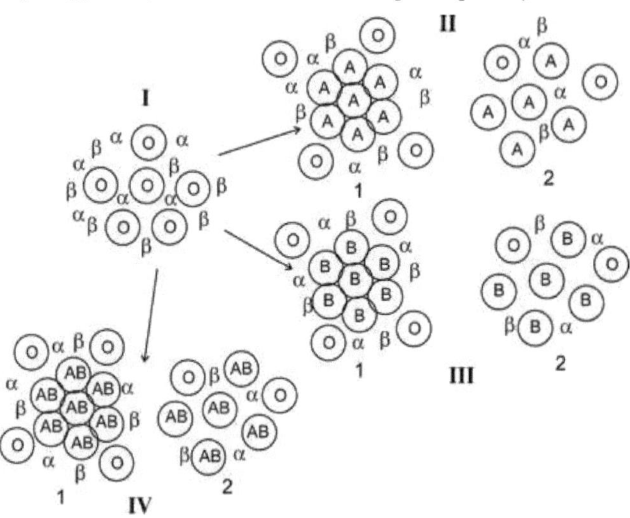

Fig.27

When group I blood (a - donor) is added to a recipient with group III blood (c), there may or may not be an agglutination reaction of the recipient's red blood cells (1).

This depends on the amount of group I blood that is added to the recipient. When group I blood is added to a recipient with group III blood, the danger is agglutinins beta in the donor's blood, which can promote agglutination of the recipient's erythrocytes, which have agglutinogen B (meeting of agglutinogens and agglutinins of the same name: agglutinogen B meets agglutinin beta). In this case, the agglutination reaction depends on a sufficient concentration of agglutinins, as they, unlike agglutinogens, can be diluted in the recipient's plasma. The threshold concentration of agglutinins at which the agglutination reaction occurs corresponds to that observed at a dilution of 1:13. In the first case (c1), a large amount of group I blood was added and the concentration of alpha agglutinins in the recipient's plasma corresponds to a dilution of 1:13 or less (1:12; 1:11, etc.). In the second case (c2), a small amount of blood was added and the concentration of donor blood alpha agglutinins in the recipient's plasma corresponds to a dilution of 1:14 or more (1:15, 1:16, etc.), so there is no agglutination reaction here, although the condition of the meeting of agglutinogens and agglutinins of the same name is met (the meeting of the recipient's agglutinogen B meets the donor's agglutinin beta, which is diluted in the recipient's plasma).

When group I blood (a - donor) is added to a recipient with group IV blood (d), there may or may not be an agglutination reaction of the recipient's red blood cells (1). This depends on the amount of group I blood that is added to the recipient. When group I blood is added to a recipient with group III blood, the danger is agglutinins beta in the donor's blood, which may promote agglutination of the recipient's erythrocytes, which have agglutinogen AB (meeting of agglutinogens and agglutinins of the same name: agglutinogen AB meets agglutinins alpha and beta). In this case, the agglutination reaction depends on a sufficient concentration of agglutinins, as they, unlike agglutinogens, can be diluted in the recipient's plasma. The threshold concentration of agglutinins at which the agglutination reaction occurs corresponds to that observed at a dilution of 1:13. In the first case (d1), a large amount of group 1 blood was added and the concentration of alpha and beta agglutinins in the recipient's plasma corresponds to a dilution of 1:13 or less (1:12; 1:11, etc.). In the second case (d2), a small amount of blood was added and the concentration of donor blood alpha and beta agglutinins in recipient plasma corresponds to a dilution of 1:14 or more (1:15, 1:16, etc.), so there is no agglutinin reaction here.), so there is no agglutination reaction here, although the condition of meeting of agglutinogens and agglutinins of the same name is met (meeting of agglutinogen AB of the recipient meets with agglutinins alpha and beta of the donor, which is diluted in the plasma of the recipient).

Fig.28 shows that when adding blood group II (a - donor) in erythrocytes with agglutinogen A and in plasma agglutinin beta to recipient with group I (b) there is agglutination reaction only of donor's erythrocytes (b2) and no agglutination reaction of recipient's erythrocytes (b1). Donor erythrocytes contain agglutinogen A, which is not diluted in the recipient's blood, and the recipient has a sufficiently high concentration of agglutinin alpha, so in this case there is an agglutination reaction of donor erythrocytes. The recipient's erythrocytes do not contain agglutinogen, so there is no agglutination.

When adding blood of group II (a - donor) in the erythrocytes of which agglutinogen A and agglutinin beta in the plasma to a recipient with group III (c), there is an agglutination reaction only of the donor's erythrocytes (c2) and no agglutination reaction of the recipient's erythrocytes (c1). Donor erythrocytes contain agglutinogen A, which is not diluted in the recipient's blood, and the recipient has a sufficiently high concentration of agglutinin alpha, so in this case there is an agglutination reaction of donor erythrocytes. The recipient's erythrocytes contain agglutinogen B, and the donor's blood has agglutinin beta, but there is no agglutination reaction, therefore, a small amount of the donor's blood has been added to the recipient and the concentration of the donor's agglutinins corresponds to a dilution of 1:14 or more (1:15, 1:16, etc.), so there is no agglutination.

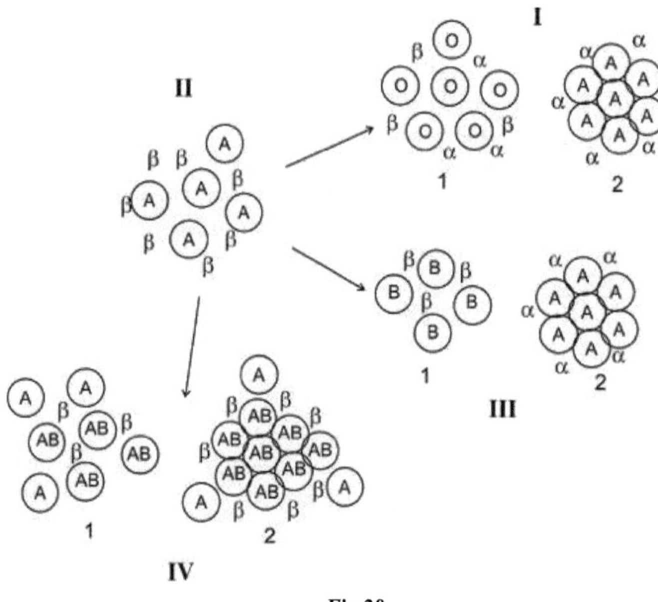

Fig.28

When adding group II blood (a - donor) with agglutinogen A in the erythrocytes and agglutinin beta in the plasma to a recipient with group IV (d), there may be an agglutination reaction of the recipient's erythrocytes (2), or there may be no agglutination reaction (1).

This depends on the amount of group II blood that is added to the recipient. When adding group II blood to a recipient with IV blood, the danger is agglutinin beta in the donor's blood, which can promote agglutination of the recipient's erythrocytes having agglutinogen B (meeting of agglutinogens and agglutinins of the same name: agglutinogen B meets agglutinin beta). In this case, the agglutination reaction depends on a threshold concentration of agglutinin beta, which, unlike agglutinogens, can be diluted in the recipient's plasma. The threshold concentration of agglutinins at which the agglutination reaction occurs corresponds to that observed at a dilution of 1:13. In

70

the second case (d2), a large amount of group 2 blood is added and the concentration of agglutinins beta in the recipient's plasma corresponds to a dilution of 1:13 or less (1:12; 1:11, etc.). In the first case (d1) a small amount of blood was added and the concentration of donor blood beta agglutinins in the recipient's plasma corresponds to a dilution of 1:14 or more (1:15, 1:16, etc.), so there is no agglutination reaction here, although the condition of the meeting of agglutinogens and agglutitinins of the same name is met (the meeting of the recipient's agglutinogen B meets the donor's agglutinin beta, which is diluted in the recipient's plasma).

Fig.29 shows that when adding blood of group III (a - donor) in erythrocytes of which agglutinogen B is agglutinin B and in plasma agglutinin alpha to the recipient with group I (b) there is agglutination reaction only of donor erythrocytes (b2) and no agglutination reaction of recipient erythrocytes (b1). Donor erythrocytes contain agglutinogen B, which is not diluted in the recipient's blood, and the recipient has a sufficiently high concentration of agglutinin beta, so in this case there is an agglutination reaction of donor erythrocytes. The recipient's erythrocytes do not contain agglutinogen, so there is no agglutination.

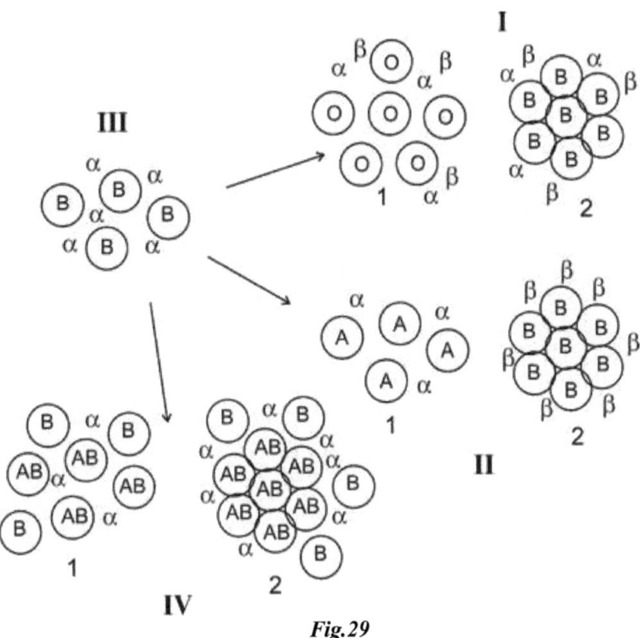

Fig.29

When adding blood of group III (a - donor) in the erythrocytes of which agglutinogen B and in the plasma agglutinin alpha to the recipient with group II (c), there is an agglutination reaction only of the donor's erythrocytes (c2) and no agglutination reaction of the recipient's erythrocytes (c1). Donor erythrocytes contain agglutinogen B, which is not diluted in the recipient's blood, and the recipient has a sufficiently high concentration of agglutinin beta, so in this case there is an agglutination reaction of donor erythrocytes. The recipient's erythrocytes contain agglutinogen A, and the donor's blood has agglutinin alpha, but there is no agglutination reaction, therefore, a small amount of donor's blood has been added to the recipient and the concentration of donor's agglutinins corresponds to dilution 1:14 or more (1:15, 1:16, etc.), so there is no agglutination.

When group III blood (a - donor) is added to a recipient with group IV blood (d), the recipient's erythrocytes may agglutinate (2) or there may be no agglutination reaction (1).

This depends on the amount of group III blood that is added to the recipient. When adding group III blood to a recipient with group IV blood, the danger is agglutinin alpha in the donor's blood, which can promote agglutination of the recipient's erythrocytes having agglutinogenes A (meeting of agglutinogenes and agglutinins of the same name: agglutinogen A meets agglutinin alpha). In this case, the agglutination reaction depends on a sufficient concentration of agglutinin alpha, which, unlike agglutinogens, can be diluted in the recipient's plasma. The threshold concentration of agglutinins at which the agglutination reaction occurs corresponds to that observed at a dilution of 1:13. In the second case (d2), a large amount of group 3 blood is added and the concentration of alpha agglutinins in the recipient's plasma corresponds to a dilution of 1:13 or less (1:12; 1:11, etc.). In the first case (d1) a small amount of blood was added and the concentration of donor blood alpha agglutinins in the recipient's plasma corresponds to a dilution of 1:14 or more (1:15, 1:16, etc.), so there is no agglutination reaction here, although the condition of meeting of agglutinogens and agglutitinins of the same name is met (the recipient's agglutinogen A meets the donor's alpha agglutinin, which is diluted in the recipient's plasma).

Fig.30 shows that when IV group blood (a-donor) with AB agglutinogen in erythrocytes and no agglutinins in plasma is added to a recipient with group I (b), only donor erythrocytes agglutinate (b2) and there is no agglutination reaction of recipient erythrocytes (b1). Donor erythrocytes contain AB agglutinogens, which are not diluted in the recipient's blood, and the recipient has a sufficiently high concentration of alpha and beta agglutinins, so in this case there is an agglutination reaction of donor erythrocytes. The recipient's erythrocytes do not contain agglutinogen, so there is no agglutination.

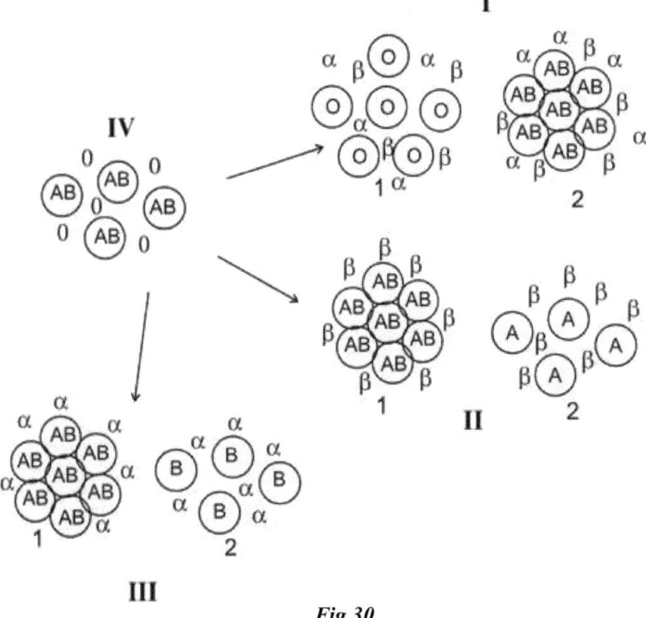

When adding blood of group IV (a - donor) in the erythrocytes of which there are AB agglutinogens and no agglutinins in the plasma to the recipient with group II (c), there is an agglutination reaction only of the donor's erythrocytes (c1) and no agglutination reaction of the recipient's erythrocytes (c2). Donor erythrocytes contain AB agglutinogens, which are not diluted in the recipient's blood, and the recipient has a high enough concentration of beta agglutinins, so in this case there is an agglutination reaction of donor erythrocytes. The recipient's erythrocytes contain agglutinogen A, and there are no agglutinins in the donor's blood, so there is no agglutination of the recipient's erythrocytes.

When adding blood of group IV (a - donor) in the erythrocytes of which agglutinogen AB is present, and in the plasma there are no agglutinins in the recipient with group III (d), agglutination reaction of the donor's erythrocytes (g1) and no agglutination reaction of the recipient's erythrocytes (g2) may occur. Donor erythrocytes contain AB agglutinogens, which are not diluted in the recipient's blood, and the recipient has a sufficiently high concentration of alpha agglutinins, so in this case there is an agglutination reaction of donor erythrocytes. The recipient's erythrocytes contain agglutinogen B, and there are no agglutinins in the donor's blood, so there is no agglutination of the recipient's erythrocytes.

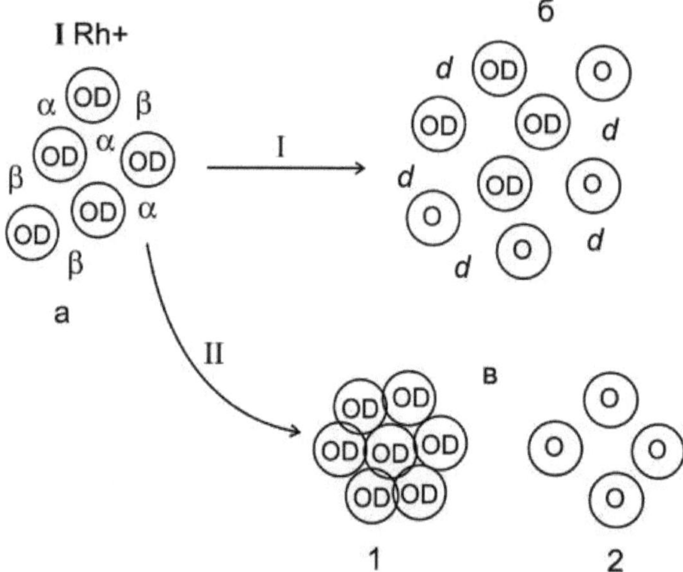

When transfusion of group I Rh positive blood (a - donor), whose erythrocytes contain D agglutinogen, to a recipient of group I but Rh negative blood (b - their erythrocytes lack D agglutinogen) occurs as follows: at the primary transfusion (I) the recipient forms d rhesus agglutinins which are not destroyed and at the secondary transfusion (II) there is agglutination of the donor's erythrocytes (1) containing D agglutinogen under the influence of d agglutinins and there is no agglutination of the recipient's erythrocytes as there is no agglutinogen in their erythrocytes.

RESPIRATORY PHYSIOLOGY

External respiration. Indicators of pulmonary ventilation. Intrapleural pressure

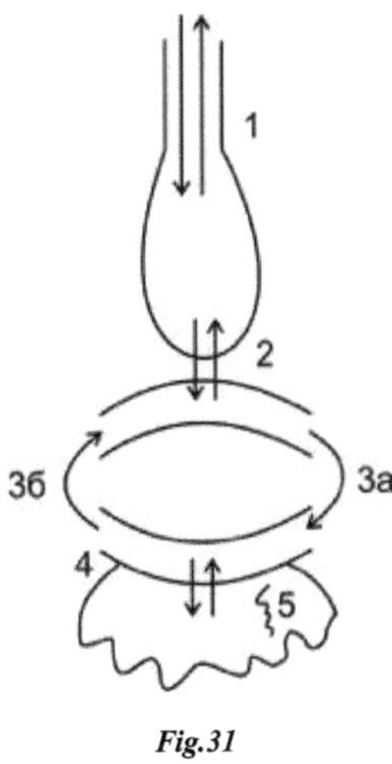

Fig.31

Fig.31 five processes occurring during respiration are marked: 1) exchange of alveolar air (A) with atmospheric air this process is called lung ventilation and is carried out due to the act of inhalation (air enters from the atmosphere into the lungs) and exhalation (exit of air from the lungs into the atmosphere); 2) gas exchange in the lungs, in which O_2 from the alveoli enters the blood, and from the blood into the alveoli enters CO_2; 3) transport of gases by the blood: O_2 is transported from the alveoli to the tissues (3a), and CO_2 is transported from the tissues to the alveoli (3b); 4) gas exchange in the tissues, in which O_2 from the blood enters the tissues, and CO_2 from the tissue enters the blood; 5) cellular respiration - due to oxidation of proteins, fats and carbohydrates.

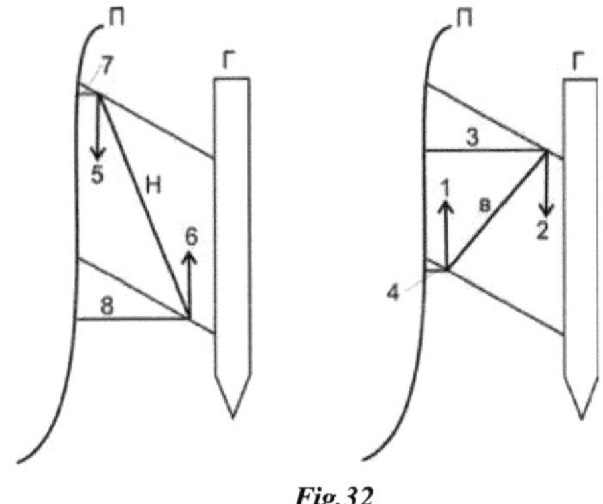

Fig.32

Figure 32 shows the mechanism of the act of inhalation (A) and deep exhalation (B) in thoracic breathing. Inhalation is an active process in which air is drawn from the atmosphere into the lungs. Active process, because it involves muscles: in thoracic type of breathing, or rib type in the act of inhalation involves the external intercostal muscle (H), in abdominal type, or diaphragmatic - involves the diaphragm, in mixed type - the external intercostal muscle and diaphragm. Figure A shows the mechanism of inhalation with the participation of the external intercostal muscle (H). When this muscle contracts, two forces act on the ribs: one force contributes to lowering the ribs (5) and the other to raising the ribs (6). These forces are equal, but the shoulder of the force that lowers the rib (7) is smaller than the shoulder of the force that raises the rib (8), so when the external intercostal muscle is contracted, the ribs rise, the volume of the rib cage increases, the intrapleural pressure decreases, the lungs stretch, the intraalveolar pressure decreases and air from the atmosphere enters the lungs - there is a breath. Calm exhalation is a passive process, as no muscles are involved. Deep exhalation is active because muscles are involved. Figure B shows the mechanism of deep exhalation with the involvement of the internal intercostal muscles (c). When this muscle is contracted, two forces act on the ribs: one force favours the lowering of the ribs (2) and the other the raising of the ribs (1). These forces are equal, but the shoulder of the force that lowers the rib (3) is greater than the shoulder of the force that raises the rib (4), so when the internal intercostal muscle is contracted, the ribs are maximally lowered, the volume of the rib cage is maximally reduced, the intrapleural pressure increases, the lungs are maximally compressed, the intraalveolar pressure is maximally increased and the maximum amount of air leaves the lungs into the atmosphere - a deep exhalation occurs.

Figure 33 shows the mechan- ism of inhalation in abdominal, or diaphragmatic, type of breathing. When the diaphragm contracts, the dome of the diaphragm decreases and the volume of the thorax increases in the vertical plane, the intrapleural pressure decreases, lung distension increases, the intra-alveolar pressure decreases, and air from the atmosphere enters the lungs - inspiration occurs.

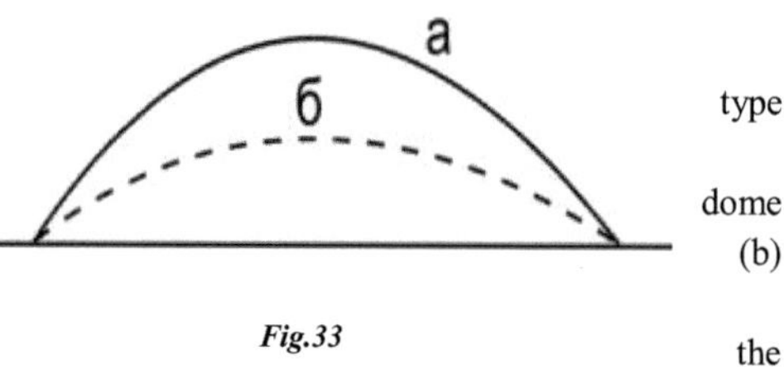

Fig.33

Fig.34 shows a spirogram (record of breathing) at rest (a, c - spirogram is recorded at a speed of 50 mm/min; b, d - spirogram is recorded at a speed of 600 mm/min), at hyperventilation (maximum deep and frequent breathing - c) and at forced exhalation (after deep inhalation a person exhales all the air as quickly as possible, the record is made at a speed of 600 mm/min - d). On this spirogram it is possible to

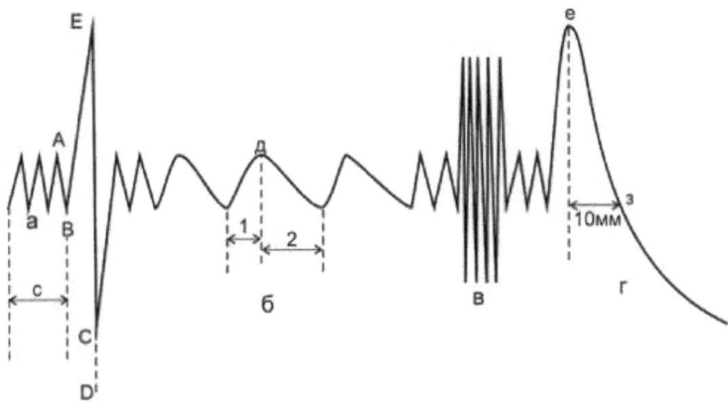

determine the following indices of pulmonary ventilation: I. Lung volumes - 1) respiratory volume (RV), the amount of air that enters the lungs during a calm inhalation, on the spirogram corresponds to AB (1mm of height corresponds to 40ml of air), in the norm RV varies between 500-800ml; 2) reserve inspiratory volume (ROVd), the amount of air that can be maximally inhaled after a calm inhalation, on the spirogram corresponds to AE, in the norm 1,5 - 2l; 3) reserve exhalation volume, the amount of air that can be maximally exhaled after a calm exhalation (ROvd), on the spirogram corresponds to BC, in the norm 1,5 - 2l; 4) residual volume (RV), the amount of air that remains in the lungs after the maximum deep exhalation. This volume does not participate in ventilation, so it is not reflected on the spirogram (marked by dotted line - CD). Thus, only three of the four lung volumes can be determined on the spirogram. II. Lung capacities - 1) vital lung capacity (VLC), consists of three volumes (DO, ROvd, ROvd), on the spirogram corresponds to EC; 2) inspiratory capacity (EFd), includes two lung volumes (DO, ROvd), on the spirogram corresponds to EF; 3) functional residual lung capacity (FoEL), includes two lung volumes (ROvd, RO), it is not determined on spirogram, as it includes OL; 4) total lung capacity (TLC), includes all four lung volumes (DO, ROvd, ROvd, OL), it is not determined on spirogram, as this capacity includes OL. III. Respiratory rate (RR) - the number of respiratory cycles (inhalation and exhalation) in 1 min, in norm 18-20. To determine the HR on the spirogram it is necessary to measure the distance (P) at which the record is made at quiet breathing. Knowing the speed of recording spirogragram (50 mm/min) and the number of respiratory cycles at a distance P can determine the HR. IV. Minute respiratory volume (MRV) is determined by the product of HR by DO (MRV=MRxDO). V. Alveolar ventilation (AV) is determined by the product of HR per DO minus dead space (MS). MP is the volume of air that does not participate in gas exchange and is located in the airways. The normal volume of MF is 150 ml. AB is determined by the following formula: AB= HODx(DO-MP). MOD reflects lung capacity, and AV indicates the efficiency of lung function. The AV is the portion of the MOD that is involved in gas exchange: the greater the portion of the MOD involved in gas exchange, the more efficient the lung function. VI. Maximal ventilation (MV) is the greatest amount of air that can pass through the lungs when breathing as deeply and frequently as possible (hyperventilation). To determine MV, record a spirogram for 15 seconds at maximum deep and frequent breathing (c). We determine HR (by multiplying the number of respiratory cycles at section c by 4, as the spirogram at MV was recorded for 15 sec) and DO at MV, then by the formula we determine: MV=CHDxDO (at hyperventilation). VII. Time of inhalation and exhalation - we determine at quiet breathing on the spirogram recorded at a speed of 600 mm/min (b): we lower the perpendicular from the top e and determine distance 1 (inhalation time) in mm and distance 2 (exhalation time). Knowing the speed of the spirogram recording, we convert these distances (mm) into sec. VIII. Forced expiratory volume (FEV) is the volume of air exhaled by the subject for 1 sec after the deepest possible inhalation. FEV is determined on a spirogram recorded at a velocity of 600 mm/min (d). For this purpose, we lower the perpendicular from the apex e to the point g (mm). The point g should be at a distance of 10 mm (1 sec) from the spirogram (h). Multiplying the segment e-zh by 40, we find the value of VWF in ml. IX. Lung ventilation coefficient (LVC) - shows what part of alveolar air is changed to atmospheric air during quiet inhalation. In norm CLV=1/7-1/8, i.e. at quiet inhalation only seventh (eighth) part of alveolar air changes to atmospheric air. CLV is calculated by the formula: CLV= (DO-MP)/FOEL. In this case, DO and Rovyd are determined by the spirogram, and the values of MF and PO are taken as the norm, respectively, 150 ml and 1.5 litres.

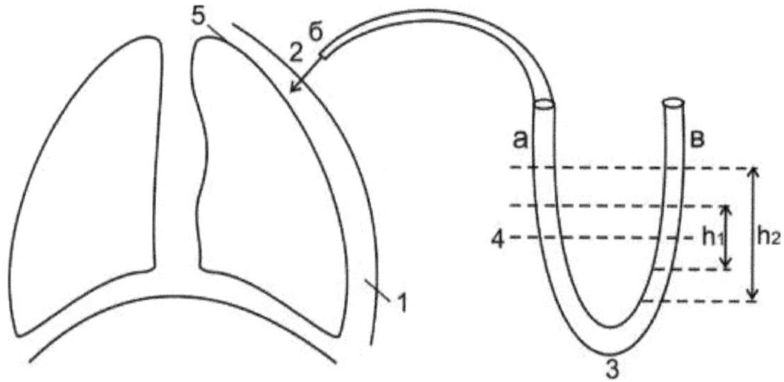

Fig.35

Fig.35 shows a method of determining the pressure in the pleural cavity (1) - a slit-like space between the visceral (5) and parietal (2) sheets of pleura. For this purpose, a U-shaped manometer (3) is used, which is filled to a certain level with water - one knee of the manometer (a) is connected to a rubber tube, the end of which is connected to a hollow needle (b). The other elbow (c) communicates with the atmosphere. Before insertion of the hollow needle into the pleural cavity (1), the water in both elbows is at the same level (zero level corresponding to the value of atmospheric pressure - 4). After insertion of the hollow needle into the pleural cavity, the water level in the manometer in knee a (connected to the pleural cavity) rises, indicating that the pressure in the pleural cavity is lower than atmospheric (negative). This pressure varies with the act of inhalation (-9 mmHg - h2) and exhalation (-5 mmHg - h2). Thus, the pressure in the pleural cavity decreases during inhalation and increases during exhalation. In both cases, the pressure in the pleural cavity is negative, i.e. below atmospheric pressure. The decrease of pressure in the pleural cavity during inhalation (-9 mmHg) in comparison with the act of exhalation (-5 mmHg) is due to changes in the elastic pull of the lungs: during inhalation (lung stretching) the elastic pull of the lungs increases the pressure in the pleural cavity decreases to -9 mmHg, and during exhalation (lung compression) the elastic pull of the lungs decreases and the pressure in the pleural cavity increases to -5 mmHg.

Blood gases. Gas exchange in lungs and tissues. Oxyhaemoglobin dissociation curve

	O_2		CO_2	
	кол-во/л (мл/л)	P (мм.рт.ст)	кол-во/л (мл/л)	P (мм.рт.ст)
Арт	200	100	520	40
Вен	120	40	580	48

This table shows the change in O2 and CO2 in arterial (Art) and venous (Ven) blood. The amount of O2 and CO2 is measured in ml per 1 litre of blood. As can be seen from the table, the amount of CO2 is significantly greater than the amount of O2 in arterial and venous blood. However, the amount of CO2 becomes greater in venous blood than in arterial blood and the amount of O2 decreases. The O2 tension (P is the pressure of O2 dissolved in blood) in arterial blood is greater than that of O2. In venous blood, RO2 decreases compared to arterial blood, and PCO2 increases.

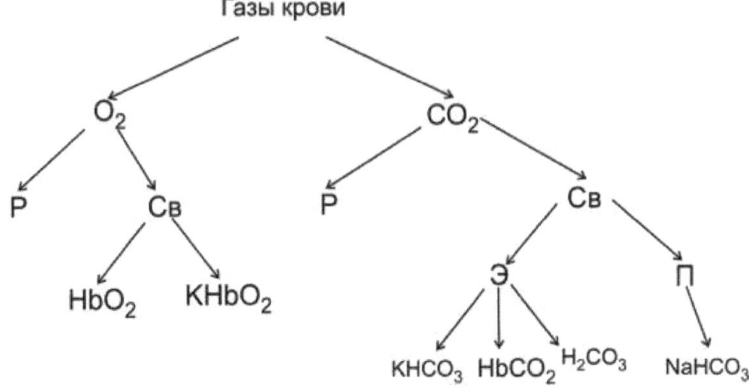

Scheme 3

Diagram 3 shows the form of CO2 and O2 in the blood. Both gases in the blood are in dissolved and bound states. O2 is dissolved (P) in plasma (0.3% of the total) and bound (Cv) in red blood cells (99.7%) as oxyhaemoglobin (HvO2) and the potassium salt of oxyhaemoglobin (KNvO2). CO2 is also in the dissolved state (2.5%) in plasma and bound state in plasma (P) and erythrocytes (E). In plasma, CO2 is in the form of sodium bicarbonate (NaHCO3 - about 45%). In erythrocytes, CO2 is in the form of potassium bicarbonate (KHCO3 - about 45%), carbohaemoglobin (HvCO2 - 5-8%) and carbonic acid (H2CO3 - 2.5%).

Fig.36 shows the layers of the alveolar-capillary membrane (ACM) through which gas exchange in the lungs takes place: O2 (1) from the alveoli enters the blood, and CO2 (2) from the blood exits into the alveolus. The ACM consists of the following layers: alveolar membrane (3); interstitial fluid (2 - between the alveolar membrane and the capillary wall of the small circulation circle - K); capillary endothelium (4); blood plasma (6) and erythrocyte shell (7).It should be noted that the two layers of the ACM (interstitial fluid and plasma) are liquid, so the ability of gases to penetrate through the ACM is influenced by their solubility in the liquid medium: the greater the solubility of the gas in the liquid, the greater the amount of it passes through the ACM. At the capillary level of the small circle of blood circulation the following processes take place: 1) O2 from alveoli through the ACM enters the erythrocyte due to the difference

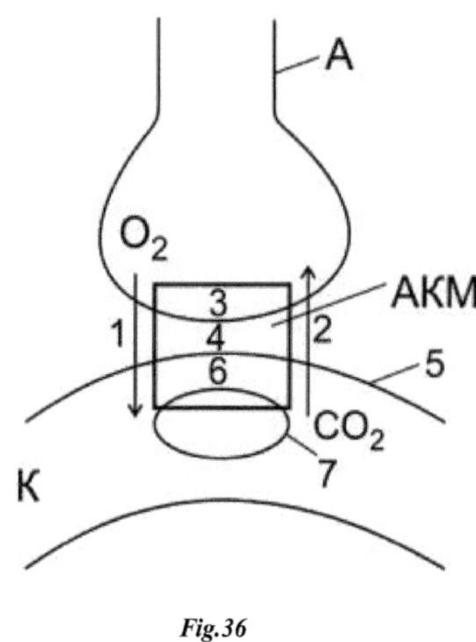

Fig.36

of partial pressure of O2 in alveolar air (100 mm Hg) and partial tension of O2 in venous blood (40 mm Hg); 2) in erythrocyte O2 is transported through the ACM to the erythrocyte due to the difference of partial pressure of O2 in alveolar air (100 mm Hg) and partial tension of O2 in venous blood (40 mm Hg).); 2) in erythrocytes due to the increase in O2 tension, its affinity for Hv increases, which leads to the decomposition of carbohaemoglobin with the formation of oxyhaemoglobin (HHvCO2 + O2 = HvO2 + CO2 + H) and the release of CO2 into the alveolus due to the difference in carbon dioxide tension in venous blood (48 mm Hg. Hg.) and alveolar air (40 mm Hg.); 3) The formed HvO2 displaces the anion HCO3 from potassium bicarbonate (HvO2 + KHCO3 = KHvO2 + HCO3); 4) The formed anion HCO3 combines with H to form carbonic acid (H + HCO3 = H2CO3), which under the influence of the enzyme carboanhydrase breaks down into water and carbon dioxide, which is released from the blood into the alveolus (H2CO3 + carboanhydrase = H2O + CO2). Thus potassium bicarbonate gives up CO2 through intermediate reactions: firstly, KNCO3 gives up carbon dioxide in the form of anion HCO3, then this anion combines with hydrogen ions to form carbonic acid, which is broken down into

80

carbonic acid under the influence of carboanhydrase; 4) in the formation of anions HCO3 chlorine ions leave the erythrocyte into the plasma, where it combines with sodium bicarbonate, displacing anions HCO3 (NaHCO3 + Cl = NaCl + HCO3), which comes from the plasma into the erythrocyte, where it combines with hydrogen ions and forms carbonic acid, which under the influence of carboanhydrase decomposes into water and carbon dioxide, which is released into the alveolus. Thus, two main processes occur in the capillaries of the small circle of the circulation: I - formation of oxygen compounds (oxyhaemoglobin - HvO2 and potassium salt of oxyhaemoglobin - KNvO2); II - decomposition of carbon dioxide compounds with its subsequent release into the alveola (in plasma there is decomposition of sodium bicarbonate - NaHCO3, in erythrocytes - decomposition of carbohaemoglobin - HnvCO2 and potassium bicarbonate - KNSO3).

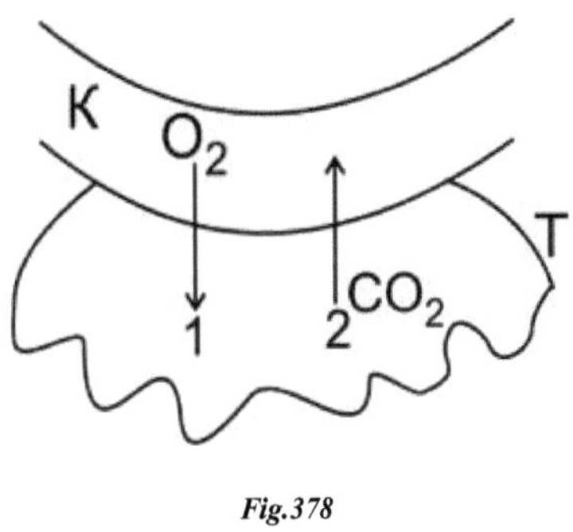

Fig.378

Figure 37 shows the process of gas exchange in tissues (T), which is carried out in capillaries of the great circle of circulation (K): O2 from the blood enters the tissues(1) due to the difference in oxygen tension between blood (100 mmHg) and tissue fluid (40 mmHg), and CO2 leaves the tissue into the blood (2) due to the difference in CO2 tension between blood (40 mmHg) and tissue fluid (48 mmHg). The following processes occur in the capillaries of the great circle of circulation: 1) CO2 penetrates from the tissue into the blood: first into the plasma, then into the erythrocyte, where under the influence of the enzyme carboanhydrase combines with water, forming carbonic acid (CO2 + H2O + carboanhydrase = H2CO3). As a result of dissociation, hydrogen cations and anions of HCO3 are formed; 2) the formed hydrogen ions reduce the affinity of haemoglobin for oxygen, which leads to the breakdown of the potassium salt of oxyhaemoglobin (KNvO2 + H = K + HHv + O2); 3) the released oxygen penetrates into tissues, potassium cation combines with anion of HCO3, forming potassium bicarbonate (K + HCO3 = KHCO3); 4) reduced haemoglobin (HHv) combines with carbon dioxide, which does not combine with water, forming carbohaemoglobin (HHv + CO2 = HHvCO2). The formation of potassium bicarbonate is limited by the presence of potassium cations (K is less than the anions of HCO3) resulting in an excess of HCO3 anions that pass into the plasma. To keep the anion concentrations between the plasma and erythrocyte at the same level, chlorine anions pass from the plasma into the erythrocyte in place of the HCO3 anions. The released sodium ion combines with HCO3 to form sodium bicarbonate (NaCl   - Na + Cl, the resulting chlorine penetrates into the erythrocyte to replace the incoming anion HCO3 from the erythrocyte; Na + HCO3 = NaHCO3). Thus, two main processes occur in the capillaries of the great circle of circulation: I - formation of carbon dioxide compounds: in plasma sodium bicarbonate (NaHCO3), and in erythrocytes carbonic acid (H2CO3), potassium bicarbonate (KNCO3) and carbohaemoglobin (HHvCO2); II - breakdown of the potassium salt of oxyhaemoglobin (KNvO2).

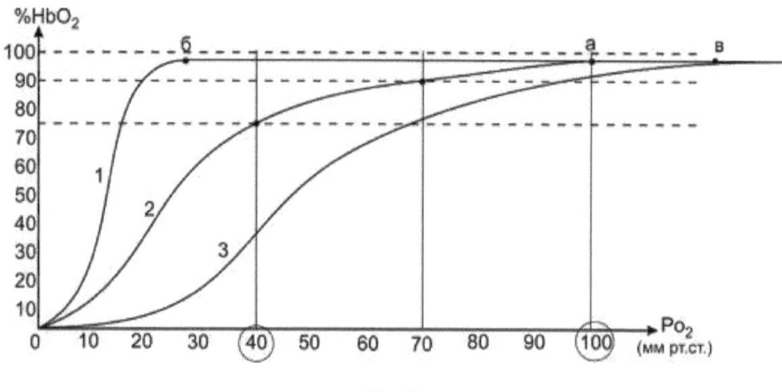

Fig.38

Figure 38 shows the oxyhaemoglobin dissociation curve, which shows the relationship between the percentage of oxyhaemoglobin (%HvO2) and the partial pressure of oxygen (PPO2).;40 mmHg is the partial pressure of oxygen in venous blood and 100 mmHg is the partial pressure of oxygen in arterial blood. - is the partial pressure of oxygen in venous blood and 100 mmHg is the partial pressure of oxygen in arterial blood. The diagram shows three oxyhaemoglobin dissociation curves: the normal curve (2), which is observed under normal conditions (at sea level, atmospheric pressure 760 mmHg.); shift of oxyhaemoglobin dissociation curve to the left (1) and to the right (2).The scheme shows that under normal conditions in venous blood (RO2=40 mm Hg) about 75% of oxyhaemoglobin is observed, and in arterial blood (RO2=100 mm Hg) the maximum saturation of haemoglobin is observed.It should be noted that 100% oxyhaemoglobin (all blood oxygen is connected with Hg) will not be present, as part of the oxygen penetrated into the blood is in dissolved form (0.3%).The shift of the dissociation curve to the left and right shows the change in the affinity of haemoglobin for oxygen. When the dissociation curve is shifted to the left (1), the affinity of Hv to oxygen increases and the point of maximum saturation of Hv with oxygen (b) is marked at RO2=55 mmHg. When the dissociation curve is shifted to the right (3), the affinity of Hv to oxygen decreases and the point of maximum shift (c) is noted at the increase of RO2 more than 100 mmHg, which can be achieved by inhalation of pure oxygen. Thus, when the oxyhaemoglobin dissociation curve shifts to the right (3), the affinity of Hv for oxygen decreases and HvO2 decays, tissues receive more oxygen (HvO2 → Hv+O2). When the oxyhaemoglobin dissociation curve is shifted to the left (1), the affinity of Hv for oxygen increases and more HvO2 is formed, tissues receive less oxygen (Hv+O2 → HvO2). The index by which the affinity of haemoglobin to oxygen is determined is called the P50 index - it is the partial pressure of oxygen at which 50% of HvO2 is formed: the higher the P50, the lower the affinity of Hv to oxygen and the less HvO2 is formed, hence tissues receive more oxygen. Five factors affect the affinity of Hv for oxygen:1)ROS2 - the greater the ROS2, the greater the affinity of Hv for oxygen (the greater the % oxyhaemoglobin formed); 2) PCO2 (carbon dioxide tension in the blood)- the greater the PCO2, the less the affinity of Hv for oxygen (the less the % HvO2 formed); 3) blood pH (blood hydrogen index)- the greater the pH (alkalosis phenomena), the greater the affinity of Hv for oxygen (the greater the % HvO2 formed). As blood pH decreases (acidosis phenomena) Hv affinity to oxygen decreases and HvO2 decays, less % HvO2 is formed; 4) body temperature - the higher the temperature, the lower the Hv affinity to oxygen (the less % HvO2 is formed); 5) 2,3 diphosphoglycerate (2,3DPG - a product of erythrocyte membrane metabolism, which occurs when blood ROS2 decreases, this substance decreases Hv affinity to O2 and oxyhaemoglobin breaks down) - the more 2,3DPG, the less Hv affinity to oxygen (the less % HvO2 is formed).

Respiratory regulation

Figure 39 shows the connection of the alpha motoneuron of the diaphragm, localised in the anterior horns of the spinal cord (2) of the 3-5 cervical segments (1), with the diaphragm (4-5) via the efferent nerve (3). Impulses going along the efferent nerve contribute to the contraction of the diaphragm, the dome of which

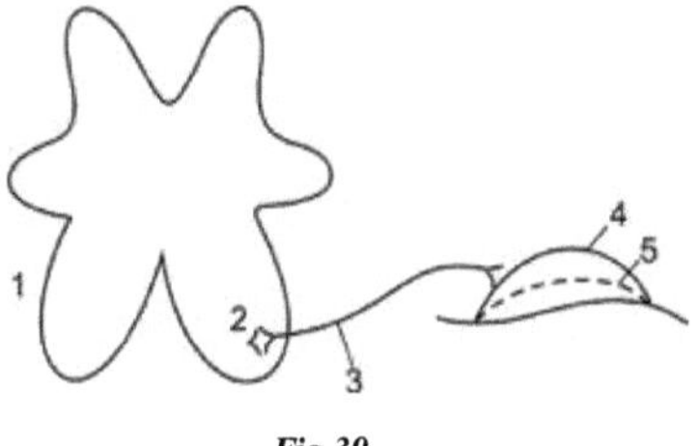

Fig.39

flattens (5) and the act of breathing in the abdominal (diaphragmatic) type of breathing occurs. When the diaphragm relaxes, its dome enlarges (4) and the act of exhalation occurs.

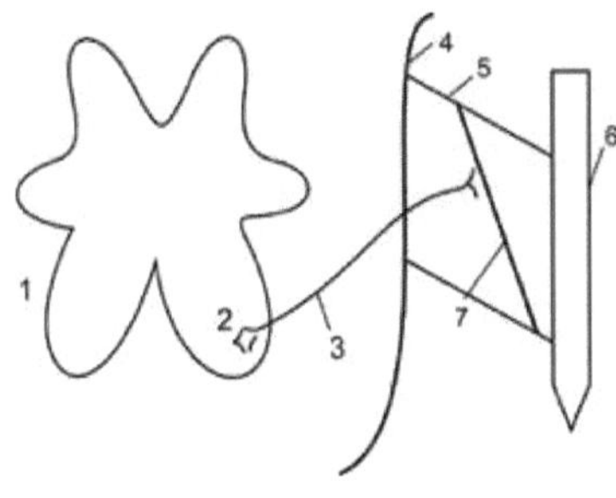

Fig.40

Figure 40 shows the connection of the alpha motoneuron of the external intercostal muscle, localised in the anterior horns of the spinal cord (2) of the thoracic segments (1), with the external intercostal muscle (7) via the efferent nerve (3). Impulses travelling along the efferent nerve promote contraction of the external intercostal muscle, as a result of which the ribs rise and the act of inhalation occurs in thoracic breathing. When the external intercostal muscle relaxes, the ribs lower and the act of quiet exhalation takes place.

Fig. 41 shows the connection of the alpha motoneuron of the internal intercostal muscle, localised in the anterior horns of the spinal cord (2) of the thoracic segments (1), with the internal intercostal muscle (7) via the efferent nerve (3). Impulses travelling along the efferent nerve contribute to the contraction of the internal intercostal muscle, as a result of which the ribs are maximally lowered and the act of deep exhalation in thoracic breathing occurs.

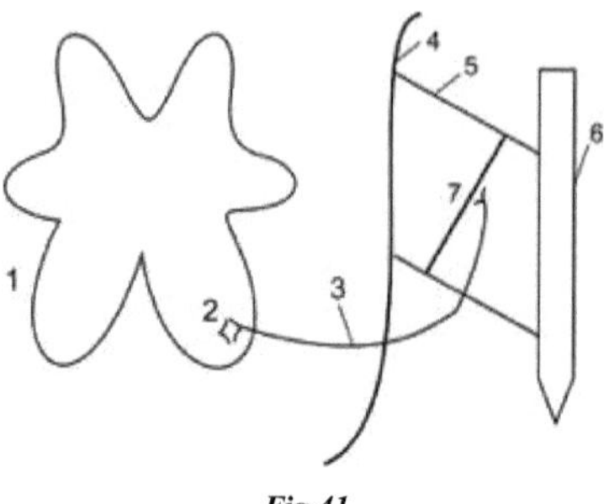

Fig.41

Fig.42 shows the connection of the alpha motoneuron of the abs (oblique and rectus abdominis muscles), localised in the anterior horns of the spinal cord (2) of the 1-2 lumbar segments (1), with the abs (4) via the efferent nerve (3). Impulses travelling along the efferent nerve contribute to the contraction of the abdominal muscles, as a result of which the intra-abdominal pressure increases and the dome of the diaphragm (5) is maximised (6), and the act of deep exhalation in the abdominal type of breathing takes place.

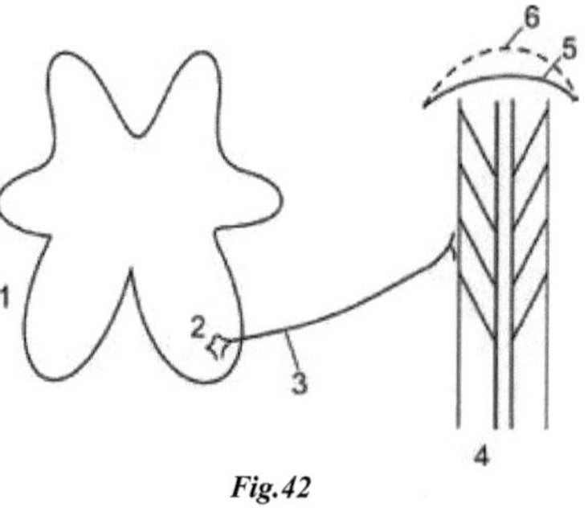

Fig.42

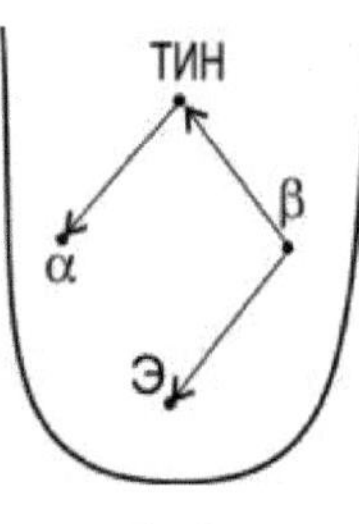

Fig.43

Figure 43 shows the localisation and composition of the respiratory centre (RC) in the medulla oblongata: TIN - inhibitory inspiratory neuron, at its excitation there is inhibition of alpha neuron and quiet exhalation is carried out; alpha neuron, at its excitation impulses through efferent pathways go to the anterior horns of either 3-5 cervical segments (here are motoneurons of diaphragm) at abdominal type of breathing, or thoracic segments (here are motoneurons of external intercostal muscles) at thoracic type of breathing and inhalation (diaphragmatic or abdominal) is carried out; beta neuron, at its weak excitation impulses go to the TIN, causing its excitation, there is inhibition of the alpha neuron and calm exhalation. At strong excitation of beta neuron impulses simultaneously go to TIN and expiratory neuron (E), causing their excitation; at excitation of expiratory neuron impulses through efferent pathways go to the anterior horns of 1-2 lumbar segments (here are motoneurons of abdominal muscles) at abdominal type of breathing, or to the anterior horns of thoracic segments (here are motoneurons of internal intercostal muscles) at thoracic type of breathing and deep exhalation is carried out.

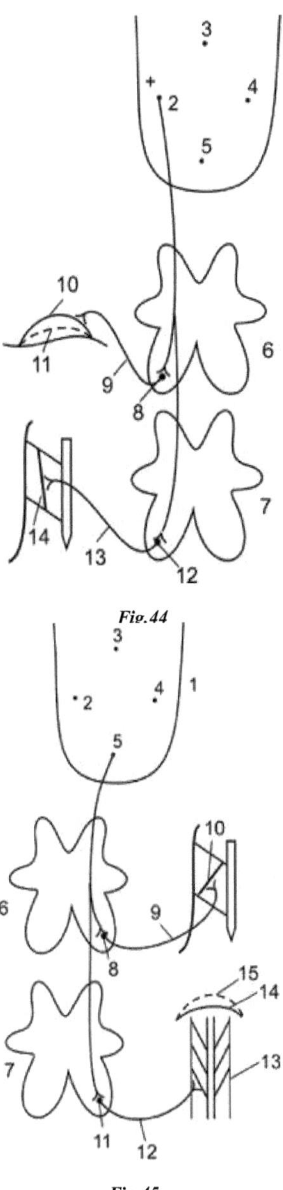

Fig.44

Fig.45

Figure 44 shows the efferent connection of the alpha neuron (2) of the respiratory centre (RC) located in the medulla oblongata (1). Impulses from the alpha neuron of the DC go to the anterior horns of the spinal cord either to the motoneurons (8) of the 3-5 cervical segments (6) in abdominal breathing, or to the motoneurons (12) of the thoracic segments in thoracic breathing, or simultaneously to 8 and 12 in mixed breathing. Impulses along the axon (9) of motoneuron (8) go to the diaphragm (10), causing its contraction (its dome flattens - 11), there is an abdominal type of breath. Impulses along the axon (13) of the motoneuron (12) go to the external intercostal muscle (14), causing its contraction; thoracic-type inspiration occurs.

Figure 45 shows the efferent connection of the expiratory neuron (5) of the respiratory centre (RC) located in the medulla oblongata (1). Impulses from the expiratory neuron of the DC go to the anterior horns of the spinal cord either to the motoneurons (8) of the thoracic segments (6) in thoracic breathing, or to the motoneurons (11) of the 1-2 lumbar segments in abdominal breathing. Impulses along the axon (9) of motoneuron (8) go to the internal intercostal muscle (10), causing its contraction, the ribs are maximally lowered, and a deep exhalation of the thoracic type occurs. Impulses along the axon (12) of the motoneuron (11) go to the abdominal muscles (13 - rectus and oblique abdominal muscles), causing their contraction, as a result, the intra-abdominal pressure increases, the dome of the diaphragm increases maximally, and deep exhalation of the abdominal type occurs.

Fig.46 shows afferent connections of alpha (1) and beta (3) neurons of the respiratory centre (RC) localised in the medulla oblongata (5). Afferent connections of the alpha neuron: 1) afferent pathway (10) from peripheral chemoreceptors (6 - PCR), the adequate stimulus of which is a decrease in oxygen tension in arterial blood; 2) afferent pathway (11) from mechanoreceptors (MR) of skeletal muscles (7), which are excited by skeletal muscle contraction, i.e. by physical exercise; 3) afferent pathway (12) from MRs of internal intercostal muscles (9), which are excited during their contraction (during deep exhalation, e.g., during physical exertion); 4) afferent pathway (13) from MRs of abdominal muscles (8). Thus, at rest, impulses to alpha neurons come from the PCP. Impulses from MR of skeletal muscles are received only during load (warning regulation). The other pathways receive impulses in those situations when deep exhalation occurs (e.g., exertion).

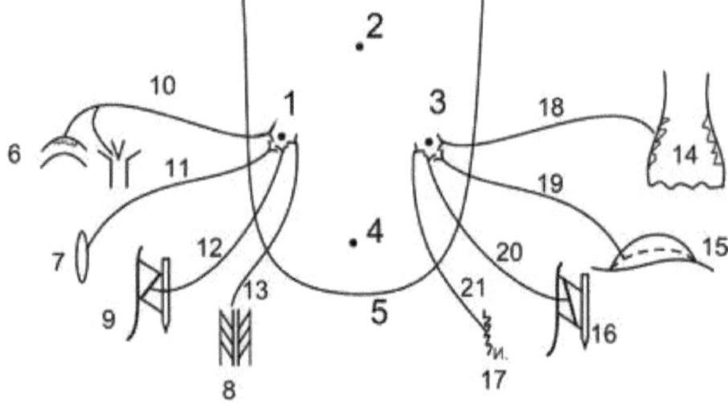

Fig.46

Impulses travelling along all pathways contribute to the excitation of alpha neurons. It should be noted that excitation of alpha neuron also occurs at irritation of central chemoreceptors localised on the lateral surface of the medulla oblongata, the adequate stimulus of which is the increase of CO_2 tension in arterial blood. The afferent connections of the beta neuron are: 1) afferent pathway (18) from the MRs of the alveoli (14), which are excited when the alveoli are distended (during inspiration); 2) afferent pathway (19) from the MRs of the diaphragm (15), which are excited when the diaphragm contracts; 3) afferent pathway (20) from MRs of external intercostal muscles (16), which are excited during their contraction (during inhalation); 4) afferent pathway (21) from irritant receptors (17), which are located in the airways and are excited during lung collapse. When these receptors are excited, inhibition of the beta neuron occurs and a deep inhalation (sigh) is performed - and the sleeping parts of the lungs are stretched. All afferent pathways, except from irritant receptors, cause excitation of beta neurons of DC.

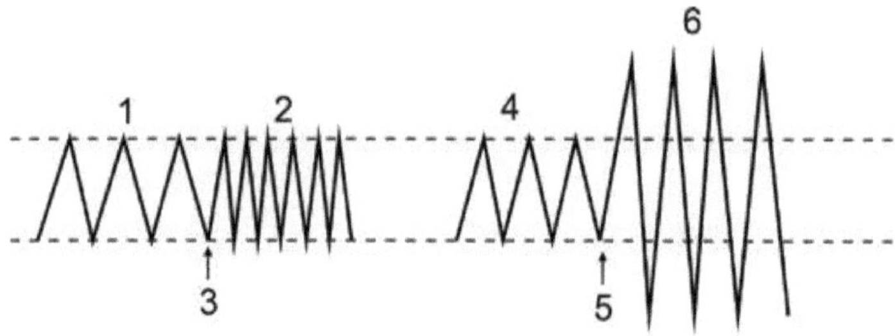

Fig.47

Fig.47 shows the spirogram at rest (1, 4 - normopnoea), at irritation of peripheral chemoreceptors (3 - PCR) due to reduction of O_2 tension in arterial blood and at irritation of central chemoreceptors (5 - CXR). The given spirogram shows peculiarities at irritation of PCR and CXR. At irritation of PCR there is (3) increase in respiratory rate (RR) without change of respiratory volume (RV) - such type of ventilation is called tachypnoeic (2). When CXR is stimulated, there is an increase in DO without a change in HR - this type of ventilation is called hyperpnoeic (6).

Fig.48 shows the spirogram at rest (1 - normopnoeic), at maximum frequency and deep breathing (2 - hyperventilation). After sufficiently prolonged hyperventilation there is an involuntary respiratory arrest (3 - apnoea) due to a sharp decrease in carbon dioxide tension in arterial blood. After apnoea there is a decrease in respiratory rate and

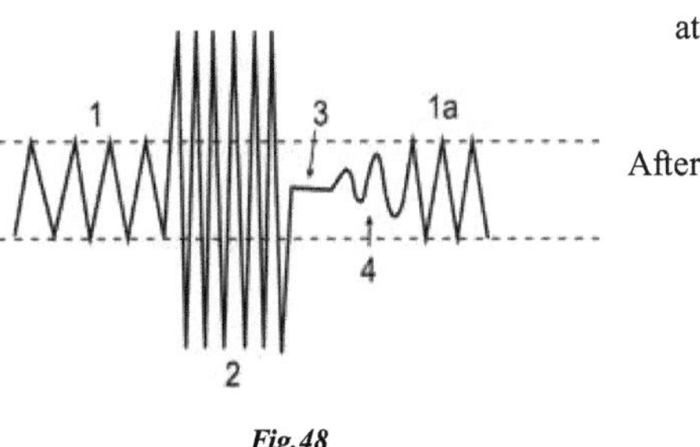

Fig.48

respiratory volume (hypoventilation). As CO2 tension in arterial blood normalises, respiratory rate and respiratory volume are restored (1a-normopnoea).

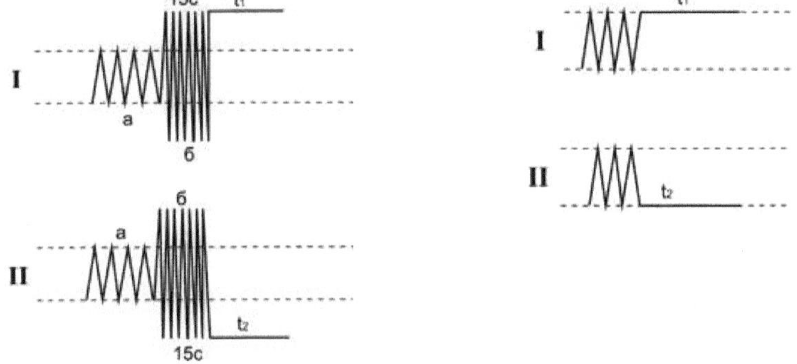

These spirograms reflect the time of maximal breath-hold in the following situations: I - time (t1) of maximum breath hold at the height of deep inhalation after 15 sec of hyperventilation (maximum deep and frequent breathing); II - time (t2) of maximum breath hold at the height of deep exhalation after 15 sec of hyperventilation; III - time (t3) of maximum breath hold during calm breathing at the height of calm inhalation; IV - time (t4) of maximum breath hold during calm breathing at the height of calm exhalation. Considering the same subject, the longest breath hold is t1, followed by t2, then t3 and the shortest breath hold is t4, which depends on the percentage of O2 and CO2 in the alveolar air: in the first case the lowest % CO2 and the highest % O2 - as we approach the fourth spirogram, % CO2 increases and % O2 falls. The lowest % O2 and the highest % CO2 is noted in the fourth case, so this situation has the shortest maximum breath-hold time. In all cases, after breath-holding, for some time (until calm breathing is restored), hyperventilation is noted. It should be noted that the respiratory rate, respiratory volume and duration of hyperventilation are the same in all cases, because in all cases at the end of breath-holding in the alveolar air at approximately the same percentage of CO2 and O2.

DIGESTIVE SYSTEM

Digestive tract research methods. Digestion in the oral cavity and stomach

Scheme of the parasympathetic nervous regulation of salivation. The salivary centre is located in the medulla oblongata (1) and consists of two sections: the upper salivary centre (2) and the lower (3). Impulses from chemo-, thermo- and mechanoreceptors of the oral cavity are sent to the salivary centre via afferent pathways. From the upper salivary centre impulses via efferent pathways arrive to the intramural ganglia of the submandibular (5) and submandibular (6) salivary glands. Acetylcholine is released in the endings of postganglionic fibres (10,11) that terminate in the hyoid (8) and submandibular (9) salivary glands. Acetylcholine interacts with the H-cholinoreactive substance and there is an

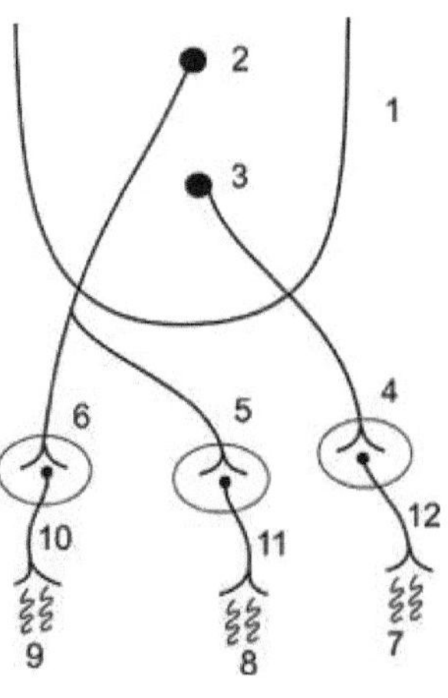

increase in the function of these glands. From the inferior salivary centre, impulses via efferent pathways enter the intramural ganglion of the parotid salivary gland (4). Acetylcholine is released at the endings of postganglionic fibres (12), which terminate at the parotid salivary gland (7). Acetylcholine interacts with the H-choline-reactive substance and the function of this gland is enhanced. Thus, at irritation of parasympathetic nerve sharply increases (10-15 times) the rate of salivation (rate of spontaneous salivation 0,5-0,7 ml/min) of liquid consistency.

Scheme of the sympathetic nerve regulation of salivary secretion. The neurons

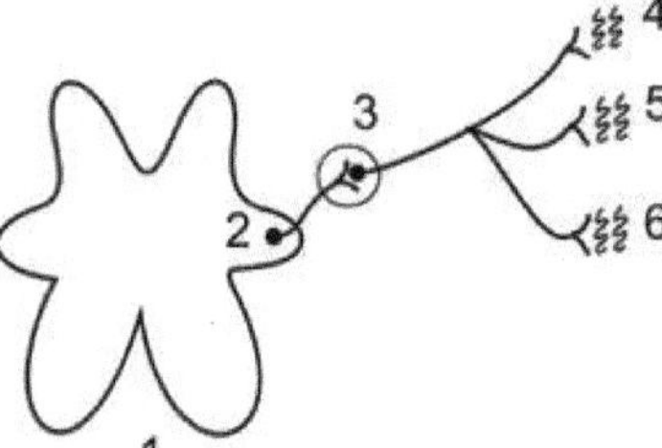

whose outgrowths form the sympathetic nerve for salivary glands are located in the lateral horns of the spinal cord of 1-2 thoracic segments (1). Acetylcholine is released in the endings of preganglionic fibres, which terminate in the paravertebral ganglion (3). Acetylcholine interacts with the H-choline-reactive substance of the postsynaptic membrane resulting in an excitatory postsynaptic potential (EPSP). In the endings of postganglionary fibres, norepinephrine is released, which interacts with the beta1 adrenoreactive substance of the postsynaptic membrane of the submandibular (4), hyoid (5) and parotid (6) salivary glands - salivary secretion rate increases only 1.5-2 times. In this case, saliva of thick consistency is secreted (due to a large amount of organic substances). Such saliva poorly moistens the oral cavity and creates a subjective feeling of dryness in the mouth.

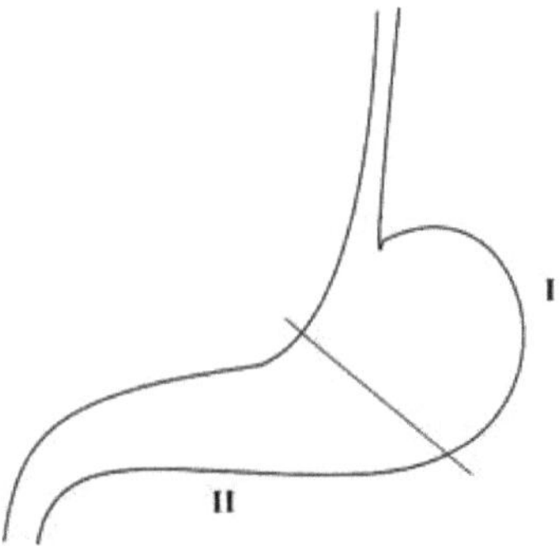

From a functional point of view, the stomach is divided into two parts: the fundic (I) and the pyloric (II). This division is due to the presence of glandular cells. In the fundal part of the stomach there are three types of glandular cells: 1) main cells, which secrete gastric juice enzymes; 2) supplementary cells, which secrete mucoid mucus; 3) lining cells, which contribute to the secretion of hydrochloric acid. In the cytoplasm of the lining cells there is an enzyme carboanhydrase due to which in these cells carbonic acid (CO_2 + H_2O = H_2CO_3) is formed, which dissociates into hydrogen cation and anion HCO_3. The hydrogen cation is released into the gastric cavity, combines with the chlorine anion and hydrochloric acid is formed. There are no lining cells in the pyloric part of the stomach, so no hydrochloric acid is formed in this part of the stomach. Thus the gastric juice of the fundal part is more acidic (pH= 0.7 to 3.0), while in the pyloric part it is less acidic (pH=5-6).

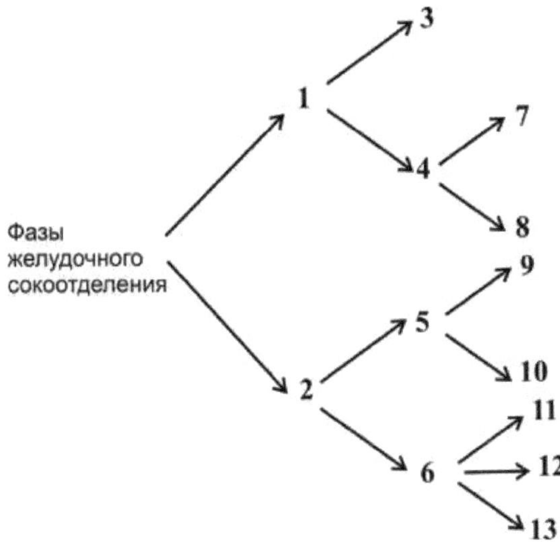

The regulation of gastric juice secretion is carried out in two phases: complex-reflex phase (1) and neurohumoral phase (2). The complex-reflex phase is based on conditioned (3) and unconditioned (4) reflexes. Conditionally reflexive gastric juicing is carried out with the obligatory participation of the cortex of the large hemispheres before food enters the oral cavity. Gastric juice secretion due to unconditional reflexes is performed by irritation of chemo-, thermo- and mechanoreceptors of the oral cavity (7) and stomach (8). The gastric juice, which is secreted before the food clump enters the stomach (3,4,7), I.P. Pavlov called appetitive, or zapal. The physiological significance of this juice is to prepare the stomach for food intake and its further digestion. The neurohumoral phase of gastric juice secretion consists of two phases: gastric (5) and intestinal (6). The gastric phase (5) is fuelled by gastric hormones: histamine (9) and gastrin (10). Histamine, entering the bloodstream, humourally increases the function of the lining cells. This increases the formation of hydrochloric acid and decreases the pH of gastric juice. Gastrin, entering the blood, humoral increases the function of the main cells. At the same time, the formation of gastric juice enzymes is increased. The intestinal phase (6) begins after chyme (a mixture of food and gastric juice) enters the 12th colon due to the homones secretin (11), enterogastrin (12) and enterogastrone (13). Secretin is formed from pro-secretin by the action of hydrochloric acid on it, which enters with the chyme from the stomach into the 12th intestine. Secretin, entering the bloodstream, humourally inhibits the function of the lining cells (decreases the formation of hydrochloric acid and the pH of gastric juice increases) and increases the formation of sodium bicarbonate in the pancreas. Enterogastrin, entering the blood, similarly to gastrin, enhances the function of the principal cells, increases the formation of enzymes. Enterogastrin, entering the blood, humourally inhibits the function of main cells.

One of the ways to study the composition and properties of gastric juice is the experience of sham feeding. This method is performed through two operations: esophagotomy (oesophageal incision - 1) and gastric fistula according to Basov (2). When food is eaten in such a dog, it does not enter the stomach (the oesophagus is closed - 3) and falls out (4), and gastric juice is secreted in the stomach due to a complex reflex phase. In this method it is possible to obtain pure gastric juice (5) through the fistula.

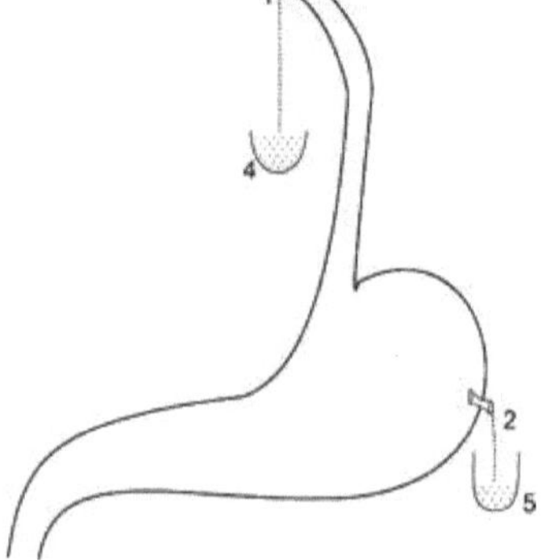

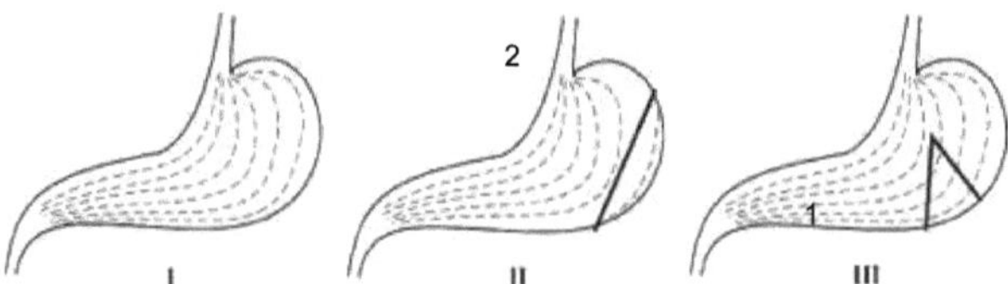

In these figures the dotted line shows the direction of the branches of the vagus (secretory) nerve. The experiment of sham feeding makes it possible to obtain pure gastric juice, but it is impossible to study the features of humoral regulation of gastric juice secretion. To study the humoral phase of gastric juice secretion, the German physiologist R. Heidengain proposed the operation of the isolated ventricle, which was modified by I.P. Pavlov. In the operation according to R. Heidengain (III), to obtain an isolated ventricle, a triangular gastric incision was made (1). I.P. Pavlov made a longitudinal incision (2) to obtain an isolated ventricle (II). Thus, the innervation of the isolated ventricle according to R. Heidengain is impaired in the isolated ventricle. This method allows to study only the humoral phase of gastric juice secretion and it is impossible to study the complex-reflex phase due to denervation of the isolated ventricle. In case of isolated ventricle according to I.P. Pavlov, it is possible to study all phases of gastric juice secretion, as the innervation of the isolated ventricle is not disturbed.

Motor and suction
digestive function

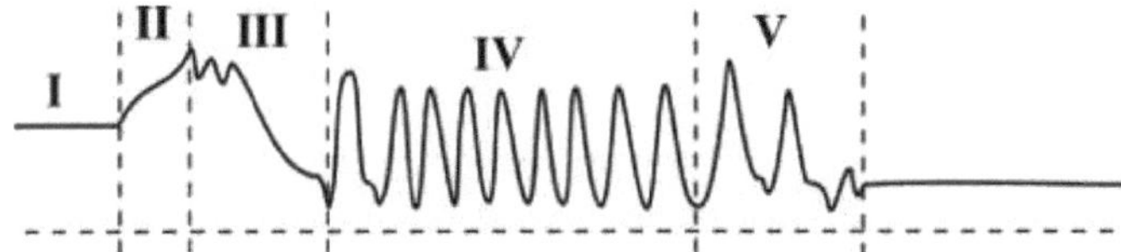

This diagram shows the registration of the biomechanics of the masticatory act (Masticaciography), which registers the change in air pressure in a rubber cuff fixed under the lower jaw. There are 5 phases on the masticatiogram: 1 phase - resting phase, the isoline is fixed (I); 2 phase - introduction of food into the mouth, it corresponds to the first rise in the curve (II), the height of which depends on the degree of mouth opening; 3 phase - oriometric (adaptation phase) is characterised by a descending curve (III); 4 phase - the main phase, there are uniform rises and falls of the curve, the amplitude and frequency of which depend on the consistency of food and fullness of the chewing apparatus (IV); 5 phase - formation of the food clump and swallowing of food (V). By the nature of the masticatory syndrome it is possible to judge about the changes in the masticatory system, about the effectiveness of orthopaedic and other therapeutic measures.

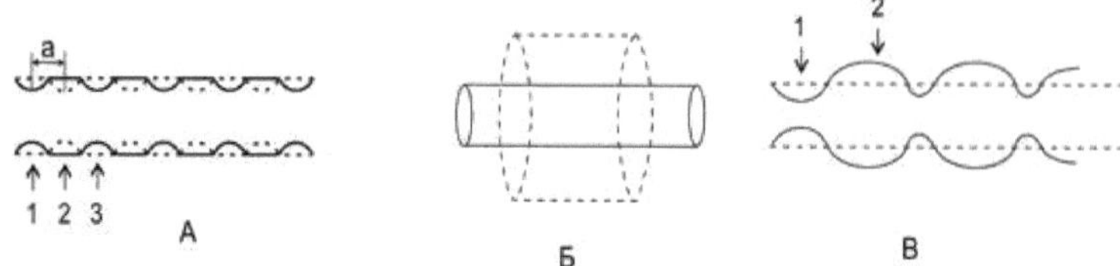

The motor function of the small intestine is performed by: rhythmic segmentation (A), pendulous movement (B) and peristaltic movement (C). Rhythmic segmentation (A) is performed by preferential contraction of only the circular muscles (1,3). As a result of periodic contraction of the circular muscles alone, a small segment of the small intestine is rhythmically divided into small (1-1.5 cm) segments (a). During rhythmic segmentation, the chyme is pulverised. The pendulous movement (B) is mainly due to the contraction of the longitudinal muscles only, which mixes the chyme with the intestinal juice. Peristaltic movement (C) is due to the coordinated contraction of circular and longitudinal muscles: circular muscles contract above the chyme, while longitudinal muscles contract below, thus moving the chyme along the digestive tract.

The diagram shows the stages of fat absorption. In the intestinal cavity, fat is broken down into glycerol and fatty acids under the influence of the enzyme lipase. Glycerol is well soluble in water and is self-absorbed. Fatty acids do not dissolve in water -

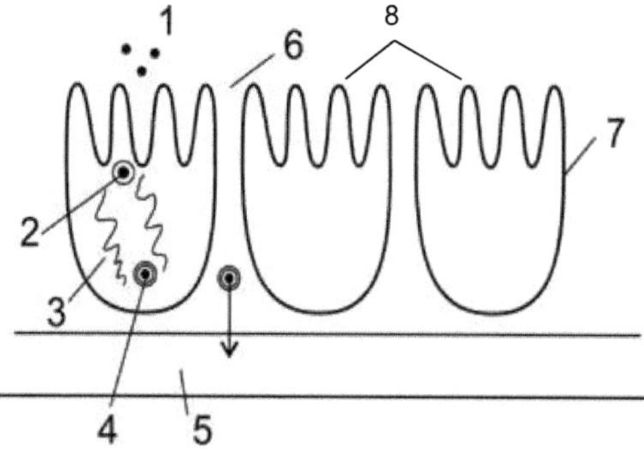

they are absorbed with the help of bile acids. The first stage of fat absorption occurs by penetration of fatty acids through the enterocyte membrane (7). The fatty acids in the intestinal cavity (1) combine with bile and are delivered to the membrane of the enterocyte apex (8). Here, the fatty acids pass through the enterocyte membrane and are converted into triglycerides (2). The second step involves the passage of triglyceride through the enterocyte endoplasmic network (3) and conversion of triglyceride into chylomicron (4 - a complex of triglycerides, carbohydrates and phospholipids). In the third step, there is penetration of chylomicron from the enterocyte cytoplasm into the intercellular space (6). In the fourth step, chylomicron penetrates from the intercellular space into lymphatic capillaries (5).

Depending on the localisation of the digestion process, a distinction is made between intracellular and extracellular digestion. In the human body, intracellular digestion takes place in neutrophils and lymphocytes. Extracellular digestion takes place in the digestive tract. There

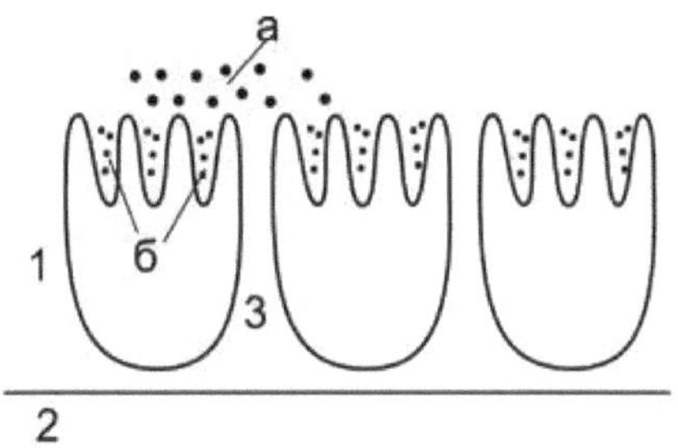

are two types of extracellular digestion: 1) cavity or distant (a) and wall or contact (b). Cavity digestion (a) is carried out at the expense of enzymes in the cavity of the digestive tract, that is, at a considerable distance from the site of enzyme formation, so this type of digestion is also called distant. The wall digestion (b) is carried out on the surface of the membrane, i.e. at contact of chyme with the membrane of enterocyte, therefore this type of digestion is also called contact digestion.

METABOLISM, THERMOREGULATION, EXCRETORY ORGANS AND ENDOCRINE SYSTEM

Metabolism and energy

Scheme of energy transformation in the organism. The source of energy in the organism are nutrients: proteins (b), fats (g) and carbohydrates (y). When these substances are oxidised with the help of oxygen, energy is formed, part of which is dissipated (E1) - this is primary heat, and most of it (E2) is converted into ATP. When energy is needed by the organism, ATP is broken down under the influence of adenosine triphosphatase (atphase). At the same time, part of the energy generated (E3 - secondary heat) is again dissipated (lost by the organism), and most of it in the form of free energy (E4) is utilised by the organism. The free energy is used for basic metabolism (WM) and work gain (WG). OE is the portion of free energy that the body expends under three standard conditions: on an empty stomach (12-14 hours after the last meal), at muscle rest (20-30 min after a horizontal position on a couch) and at a comfort temperature, i.e. in the laboratory where OE is determined, the temperature should be +20+22 degrees Celsius. The AO energy is spent on the act of breathing (contraction of muscles involved in the act of breathing - e), heart ventricular systole (c), processes occurring in the nephron (n) and liver (p), as well as on assimilation processes (ass) occurring in all living tissues. The energy of the labour augmentation is spent on: 1) the specific dynamic action of food (SDDP), i.e. the assimilation of nutrients. For the assimilation of proteins, the organism spends 30% of GS energy, fats - 12-15% and carbohydrates - 4-5%; 2) physical efficiency (PE) - any type of physical activity; 3) mental efficiency - any type of intellectual activity. Thus, the energy formed in the body can be divided into two types: 1) bound energy (primary and secondary heat) - this energy cannot be used by the organism, it is dissipated; 2) free energy (PA and RP), which the organism uses in the process of its vital activity.

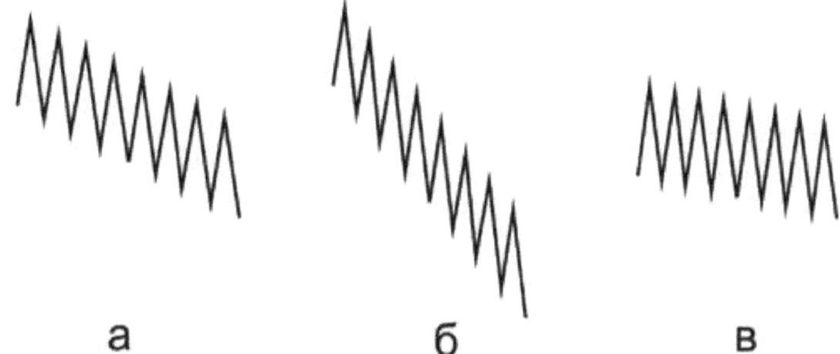

Scheme showing one of the ways to determine the energy expenditure of the organism (indirect calorimetry) at rest (c) and when performing a load of different power (a,b). The energy expenditure of the organism can be determined by direct calorimetry (PC) and indirect calorimetry (IC). To determine energy expenditure using PC, a biological object is placed in a special calorimetric chamber and all types of heat released by the organism are taken into account. This method is more often used to determine the energy expenditure of small animals. In the clinic, indirect calorimetry is used, that is, the determination of energy in an indirect way. For this purpose it is necessary to determine the following indices: 1) oxygen consumption (PO2) - the more PO2, the more energy consumption of the organism. The diagram shows the determination of PO2 using the Krogh apparatus, under the dome of which oxygen is injected and a spirogram is recorded on the drum. As oxygen is used by the organism, the dome of the device is lowered and the steepness of the spirogram is used to determine PO2. Connecting the lower points of the spirogram, we get the hypotenuse of the triangle, where one straight cathetus (ordinate) shows the value of PO2, and the second straight cathetus (abscissa) shows the time during which PO2 is noted; 2) the amount of extracted CO2. After determination of these two indices we determine two more indices by calculation method: 1) respiratory coefficient (RC) - it is the ratio of extracted CO2 to the amount of PO2. BF depends on the oxidation of which nutrient is the energy expenditure of the organism: at BF=1.0 the organism oxidises carbohydrates; at BF=0.8 - oxidation of proteins; at BF=0.7 - oxidation of fats; 2) after determining BF we find the caloric equivalent of oxygen (CEA) - it is the energy that the organism releases when consuming 1 litre of oxygen. OEC depends on the nutrient oxidised in the organism: during oxidation of carbohydrates OEC=5.05 kcal (21.14 kJ); during oxidation of fats OEC=4.7 kcal (19.64 kJ); during oxidation of proteins OEC=4.6 kcal (19.2 kJ). Knowing KEK and average daily PO2 in 1min, it is possible to calculate energy consumption of an organism for 1 min (PO2 in lHKEC), multiplying the received number by 1440 (number of minutes in 1 day) we find energy consumption of an organism during one day.

Thermoregulation

Scheme of thermoregulation, which is carried out by the thermoregulation centre located in the hypothalamus (3). This centre consists of two divisions: heat transfer - T/O (4) and heat production - T/P (5). These two departments are in reciprocal dependence: excitation of T/O results in inhibition of T/P and vice versa. Each department of the thermoregulation centre is connected with the corresponding working organs: T/O department with the

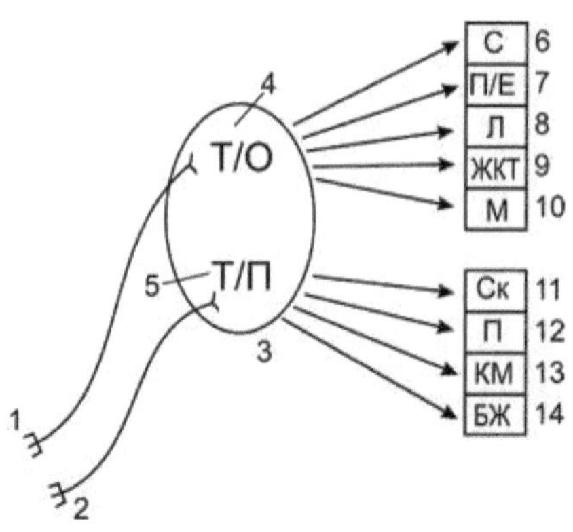

organs of heat dissipation, which increase the body's heat output and preserve it from overheating; T/P department with the organs of heat production, which increase the formation of heat in the body and preserve it from overcooling. In the body there are 4 ways of heat transfer: 1) heat conduction - this method is carried out by direct contact of the body with an object whose temperature is lower than the body temperature - in this case, the heat from the body directly passes to warm the object; 2) convection - this method is carried out through the movement of air heated by the body (the fan increases the body's heat transfer in this method); 3) heat radiation - due to the body's emission of infrared rays; 4) evaporation - when evaporating 1 ml of water, the body loses 0.58 kcal en The organs of heat transfer include: 1) skin (82% of heat is given off through the skin). Heat transfer through the skin is realised by two mechanisms: through vascular reactions (6 - when vessels dilate, heat transfer increases due to heat conduction, convection and heat radiation, and when vessels constrict, it decreases) and the work of sweat glands (7 - due to evaporation); 2) lungs (L-8) - 13% of the body's heat is given off through the lungs due to evaporation; 3) gastrointestinal tract (GI-9) - 4% of heat is given off by the body through the gastrointestinal tract due to heat conduction to warm food; 4) urine and faeces warming (M-10) - 1% of heat is given off by the body through urine and faeces warming due to heat conduction. The organs of heat production include: 1) skeletal muscles (Sk-11) - 60% of the body's heat is generated by the contraction of skeletal muscles. Heat can be generated by involuntary muscle contraction - the body shakes. The heat that is generated by involuntary muscle contraction is called shivering thermogenesis. Heat formation can occur during arbitrary muscle contraction with the participation of the cortex of the large hemispheres (a set of arbitrary muscle contractions causes behaviour, which is accompanied by an increase in heat in the body); 2) liver (P-12) - 30% of heat is formed due to redox reactions in the liver, due to this the liver is called the biochemical kitchen of the body; cellular metabolism in organs and tissues (KM-13) - in an adult organism 10% of heat is generated by cellular metabolism in organs and tissues of our organism; 4) in newborn children, in addition to the above, the organs of heat production include brown fat (BF-14), which is located in the interscapular region and in the axilla. This fat is easily oxidised and gives heat to the body (the heat generated by oxidation of brown fat is called non-fat thermogenesis). Thus, upon irritation of thermal thermoreceptors (1), impulses via afferent pathways arrive at the T/O section of the thermoregulatory centre. When this department is excited, the T/P department is first inhibited. If necessary, impulses from the T/O department via efferent pathways go to the corresponding organs of heat dissipation - heat dissipation by the organism and its preservation from overheating is increased. When cold thermoreceptors (2) are irritated, impulses along the afferent pathways go to the T/P section of the thermoregulation centre. When this department is excited, the T/O department is inhibited first. If necessary, impulses from the T/P department via efferent pathways go to the corresponding heat-producing organs - heat production by the organism and its preservation from cooling is increased.

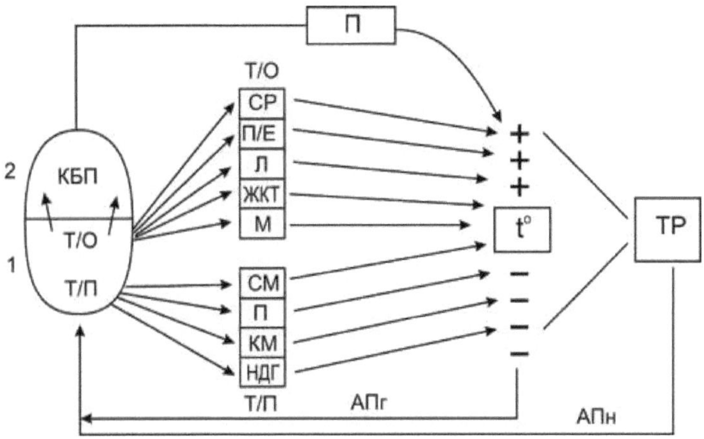

A functional system that keeps body temperature constant (t°). The first link is the final useful adaptive result - body temperature (). When body temperature changes (increase or decrease from the optimal level), the second link - specific receptors (TR - heat and cold thermoreceptors) are excited. The third link - afferent pathway: nerve (APn) from TR to CNS and humoral (APg) - in the action of blood temperature directly on the CNS. The fourth link is the CNS, in which two levels are distinguished: 1) hypothalamus (1), where the centre of thermoregulation is located, consisting of two departments - the centre of heat dissipation (T/O) and heat production (T/P); 2) the cortex of the large hemispheres (2 - HPA). Fifth link effectors: 5a are the effectors, which are divided into two groups - heat transfer organs (T/O) and heat production organs (T/P). The T/O organs include: 1) skin, where heat transfer is due to vascular reactions (SR) and sweat gland (SG) function; 2) lungs (L); 3) gastrointestinal tract (GIT); and 4) urine and faecal warming (M). The organs of the T/P include: 1) skeletal muscles (SM), which produce heat by involuntary contraction - tremor thermogenesis (VT) and by voluntary contraction involving the cerebral cortex; 2) liver (P); 3)

cellular metabolism in all organs and tissues (CM); 4) oxidation of brown fat - non-tremor thermogenesis (NTT); 5b - endocrine system, which through effectors contribute to normalisation of body temperature. The sixth (external) link is behaviour (B), which is carried out due to a set of arbitrary contractions of skeletal muscles with the participation of PMA.

EXCRETORY ORGANS

This diagram shows the processes occurring in the nephron. The first process, filtration (6), is the passage of water and some substances from the capillaries of the tubule (1) into the cavity of the Baumann-Schumlansky capsule (4). Through filtration, primary urine is formed (filtration rate up to 120 ml/min in men and up to 110 ml/min in women). The amount of primary urine per day is 150-180 litres/day. The second process is reabsorption (7), that is, the back absorption of water and some substances from the tubule cavity into the blood of the second capillary network (5). The third process is secretion (9), that is, synthesised substances in the renal tubule cells are secreted into the tubule cavity. For example, during amoniogenesis, ammonia is

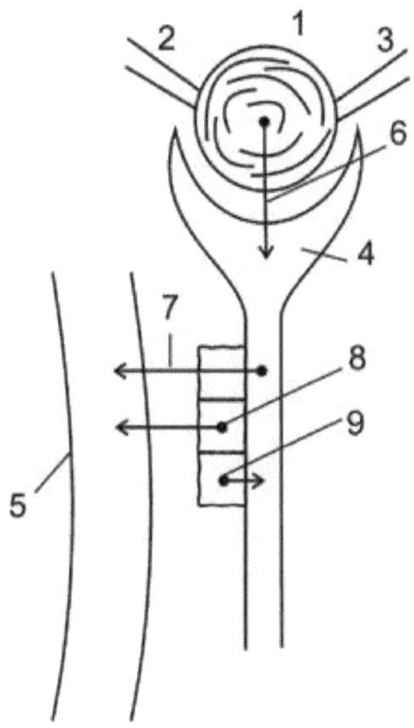

synthesised in the renal tubule cells, which captures excess hydrogen ions from the blood and ammonium is formed and excreted into the tubule cavity and further, combining with chlorine ions, is excreted with the final (secondary) urine. By reabsorption and secretion, secondary, or terminal urine is formed. From 150-180 litres of primary urine, 1.5-2 litres/day of secondary urine is formed due to reabsorption. The excreted end urine is called diuresis. A decrease in diuresis is called oliguria, absence - anuria, increase - polyuria. The fourth process - incretion (8) - synthesised substances in the cells of the renal tubules are secreted into the blood (hormonal function of the kidneys). Among these substances are: 1) haemopoietins (leuko-, erythro- and thrombopoietins), which are involved in the formation of blood forming elements; 2) renin, which converts angiotensinogen first into angiotensin I, then into angiotensin II (active vasoconstrictor), etc.

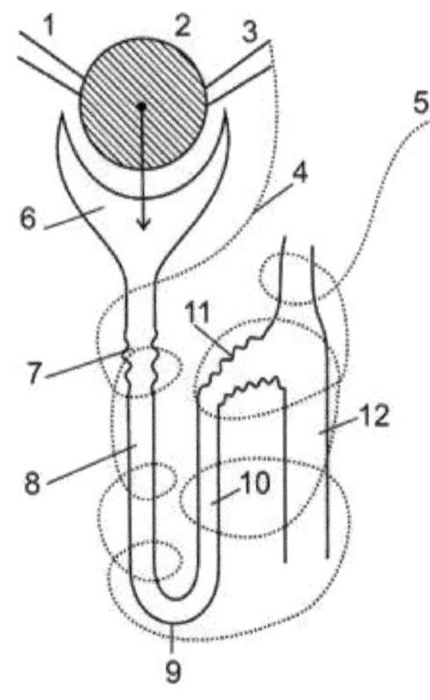

The diagram shows the structural and functional unit of the kidney - nephron: 1) bringing arteriole; 2) tubule (first capillary network); 3) bringing arteriole; 4) secondary capillary network; 5) venule; 6) Baumann-Shumlansky capsule cavity; 7) proximal convoluted tubule (first order convoluted tubule); 8) direct descending tubule; 9) loop of Henle; 10) direct ascending tubule; 11) distal convoluted tubule (second order convoluted tubule) 12) collecting tube.

MECHANISM OF ACTION OF HORMONES

The diagram shows the extracellular mechanism of action of hormones (protein, catecholamines, serotonin, histamine). Hormone action consists in activation of enzymes - protein kinase, which binds to 3,5 cyclic adenosine monophosphate (CAMP).Protein kinase consists of a regulatory subunit (P) and a catalytic subunit (K). The regulatory unit combines with CAMP, protein kinase dissociates to form a complex of CAMP with the regulatory unit (CAMP-P) and the active catalytic unit (K), which activate phosphorylation processes (f-e) and increase cell activity. At first, a hormone-protein complex is formed on the membrane surface (1), then the enzyme adenylate cyclase (A-za) is activated, and the synthesis of cAMP begins using ATP energy. This is followed by the coupling of CAMF with the regulatory unit of proetinkinase with the subsequent release of the active

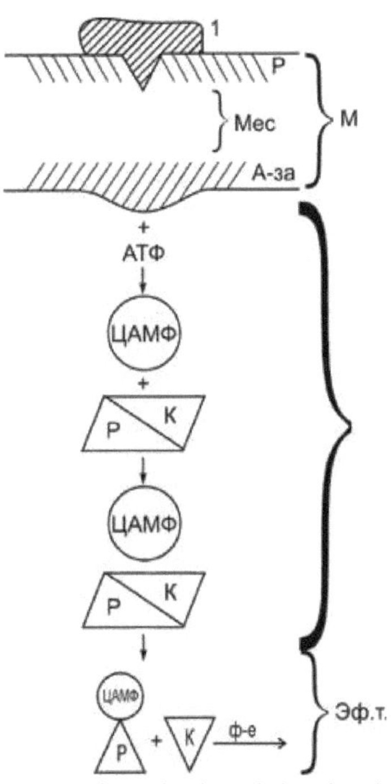

catalytic part of the protein kinase, which leads to the activation of phosphorylation processes.

The diagram shows the intracellular mechanism of hormone action (steroid hormones and thyroid hormones). The following processes take place: penetration of hormone (1) inside the cell. A hormone-carbohydrate-protein complex (2) is formed in the cytoplasm, which leads to dissociation of the complex into hormone-protein (3) and carbohydrate (6). The hormone-protein complex penetrates into the nucleus (5) and acts on chromatin filaments (4). This produces informative RNA, which promotes protein synthesis.

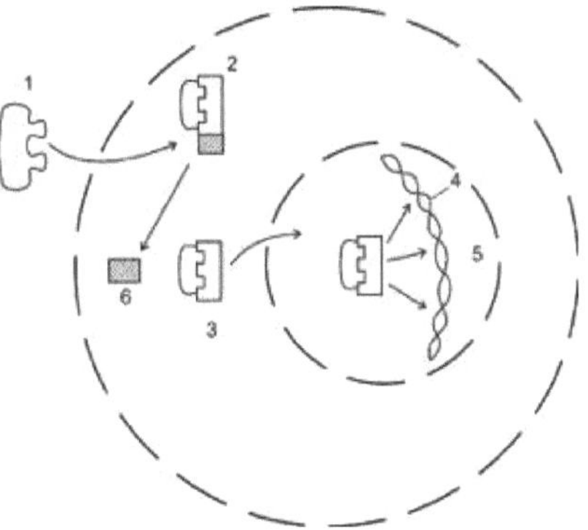

Humoral regulation of endocrine glands

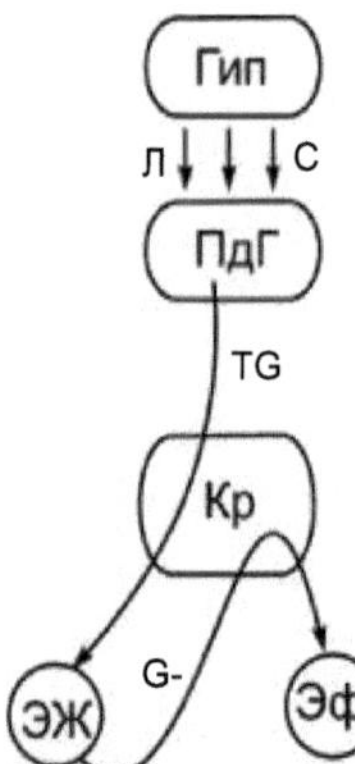

The scheme reflects the humoral mechanism of regulation of endocrine function involving the hypothalamic-pituitary system. In the hypothalamus (Hyp) liberins and statins (L, S) are formed, which through the portal system act on the anterior lobe of the pituitary gland (PdH) and enhance (liberins) or inhibit (statins) the synthesis of the corresponding tropic hormones (TH), which through the blood (Kr) act on the corresponding endocrine glands (EG), enhancing their function. The released effector hormone (G-e) affects organs and tissues by an extra- or intracellular mechanism.

This diagram shows the interaction between the hypothalamic-pituitary system and the endocrine glands. In the hypothalamus (Hyp-1) the following liberins are formed: thyreoliberin (TLB), somatoliberin (STL), corticoliberin (CLB), foliberin (FLB). All the lyberins act via the portal system on the anterior lobe of the pituitary gland (PdH - 2), where the corresponding tropic hormones are synthesised. Thyroid hormone is synthesised on the TLB (3), which acts on the thyroid gland via the blood (4). There is increased

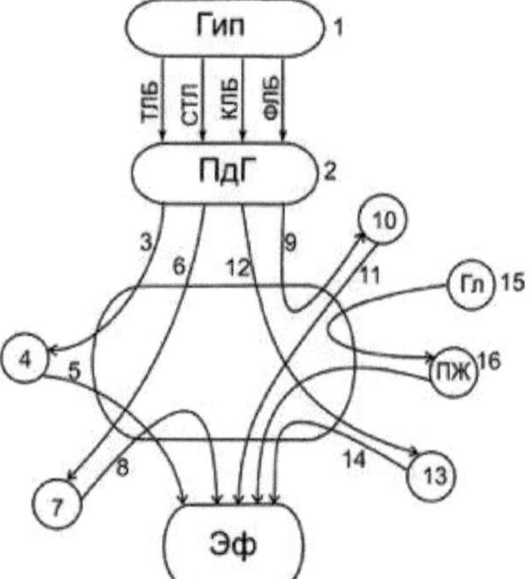

release of thyroxine and triiodothyrosine (5 - thyroid effector hormone) into the blood, which acts on organs and tissues through the blood (Eph). The STL synthesises somatotropic hormone (6), which acts on the liver(7) via the blood. There is an increased release of somatomedins (8) into the blood, which act on organs and tissues through the blood (Eph). Adrenocorticotropic hormone is synthesised on the CLB (12), which acts on the cortical layer of the adrenal glands through the blood(13). There is an increased release of corticosteroids into the blood (14), which act on organs and tissues through the blood (Eph). Follicle-stimulating hormone is synthesised on the FLB (9), which acts on the sex glands through the blood (10 - in males on the testes, in females on the ovaries). There is an increased release of androgens (in men) and estrogens (in women) into the blood, which act on organs and tissues through the blood. Increase of glucose concentration in the blood (Gl - 15) acts on the pancreas (PG - 16), insulin is released into the blood, which increases membrane permeability to glucose.

ANALYZERS

Visual

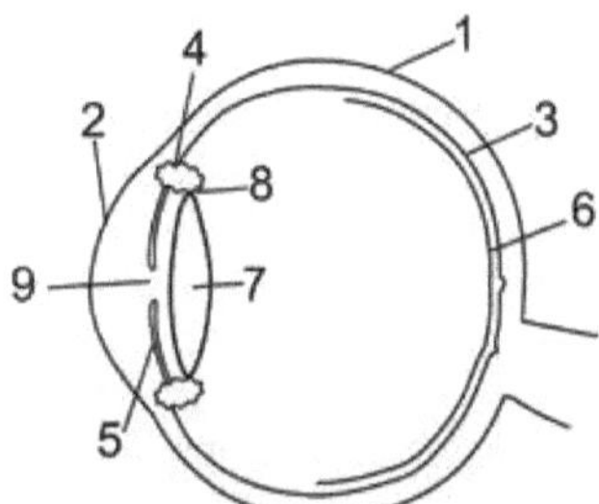

This diagram shows the three membranes of the eye: I, the outer shell, or albumen (1), which is convex and transparent in front (2) and is called the cornea (cornea); II, the middle, or vasculature (3), which is divided into three parts: The intrinsic vasculature (3), the dilated part - the accommodative muscle, or ciliary body (4) and the iris (5), which is thinned to the front and determines the colour of the eye; III - the inner, or retinal sheath (6), in which the receptor cells (rods and cones) are located. The opening in the iris is the pupil (9), which regulates the beam of light. The refractive power of the eye consists of the cornea (40 diopters) and the lens (7 - 23 diopters). Due to the elasticity of the lens and the accommodative muscle, the curvature of the lens can change: the lens becomes more convex when looking at close objects and flatter when looking at distant objects.

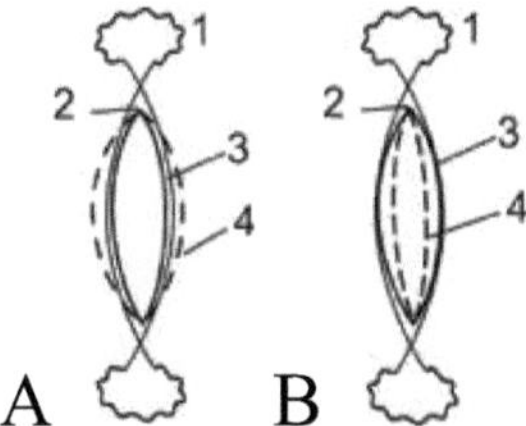

This diagram shows the mechanism of accommodation of the eye (the eye's ability to clearly see close (A) and distant (B) objects. When looking at close objects (A), there is a contraction of the accommodation muscle (1), which leads to relaxation of the cine ligament (2) and the lens (3), due to its elasticity, becomes more convex (4), the refractive power increases and the eye sees close objects clearly. When looking at distant objects (B), the acomadation muscle (1) relaxes, which leads to tension of the cine ligament (2) and the lens (3), due to its elasticity, becomes flatter (4), the refractive power decreases and the eye sees distant objects clearly.

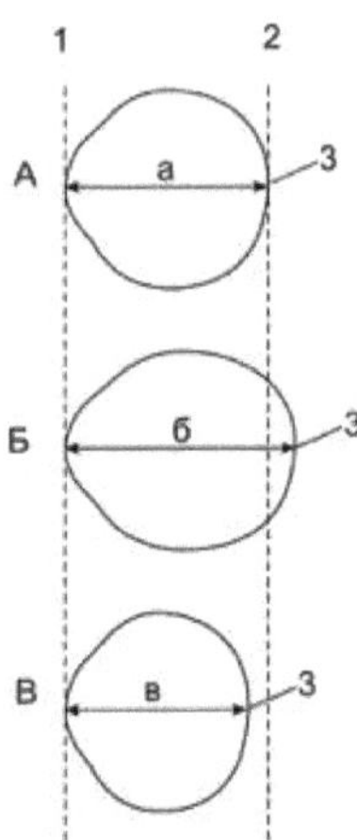

This diagram shows the normal eye, or emmetropic (A) and the types of accommodation disorders - myopic, or myopic (B) and hyperopic, or hyperopic (C). The first vertical dashed line (1) reflects the cornea of the eye. The second line (2) reflects the focal length. An accommodation disorder is detected when the accommodative muscle is completely relaxed. In a normal eye, the focus coincides with the retina (A3). In the myopic eye, the focus is in front of the retina, or closer to the retina, so this accommodation disorder is called myopia (B3), its anatomical axis is larger than in the normal eye. In hyperopic eye the focus is behind the retina, or further away from the retina, so this accommodation disorder is called hyperopia(B3), its anatomical axis is smaller than normal eye. Thus the accommodation disorder of the eye is due to changes in the anatomical axis: in myopia - the anatomical axis becomes larger than normal, and in hyperopia - smaller than normal.

This diagram shows two myopic eyes with different degrees of accommodation disorder: severe myopia (A) and less severe myopia (B). The severity of myopia is determined by the distance from the focus to the retina: the greater the distance, the more severe the myopia.

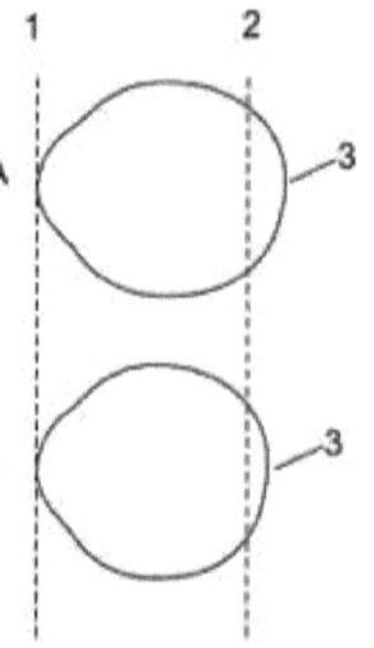

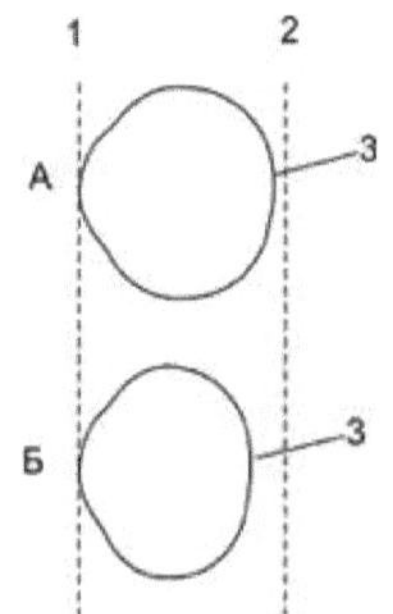

This diagram shows two hyperopic eyes with different degrees of accommodation disorder: severe hyperopia (B) and less severe hyperopia (A). The severity of hyperopia is determined by the distance from the focus to the retina: the greater the distance, the more severe the hyperopia.

This diagram shows mild myopia (A) and mild hypermetropia (B). In one of these cases a person does not experience subjective sensations of accomadation disturbance. The point is that when determining the types of accommodation disorders of the eye, the accommodation muscle is completely relaxed by injecting atropine into the eye. To correct a myopic eye, it is necessary to increase the focus, which is achieved by relaxing the accommodation muscle. Since this accomadation disorder is detected at the maximum relaxation of the ciliary body, therefore, self-correction by relaxing the muscle is impossible. This type of disorder is corrected only with the help of double-concave lenses. To correct a hyperopic eye it is necessary to reduce the focus, which is achieved by contraction of the accomadation muscle. Since this accomadation disorder is detected at maximum relaxation of the ciliary body, therefore, in case of mild hyperopia, self-correction by muscle contraction is possible. This type of disorder is corrected independently (in mild hyperopia) and with the help of double-convex lenses (in severe hyperopia)

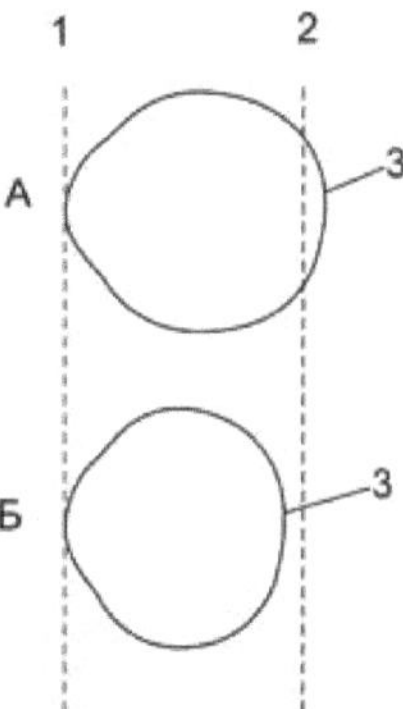

Auditory and vestibular

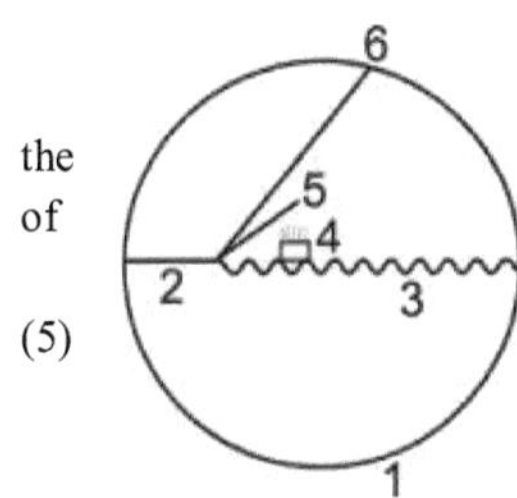

This diagram shows a transverse section of the cochlea (1). The bony ridge (2), which transitions into base membrane (3). On the base membrane is the organ Cortium (4), the receptor of the auditory analyser. At the beginning of the main membrane, the covering lamina and the Reissner's membrane branch off. When the perilymph moves, the main membrane is deformed (bent) and the hairs of receptor cells come in contact with the cover plate - an impulse arises, which reaches the temporal lobe of the cerebral cortex (Geschle's gyrus) via the auditory nerve - auditory sensations arise.

This diagram shows the inner ear, which consists of: the semicircular tubules (1,2,3), the cochlear vestibule (4,5) and the cochlea (6): base (7) and apex (8). The semicircular tubules and cochlear vestibular receptors are located in the cochlea. The cochlea contains receptors for the auditory analyser. The receptors of the semicircular tubules are represented by the hairbrush - their adequate stimulus is rotary movements. Receptors of the cochlear vestibule are represented by the otolith - their

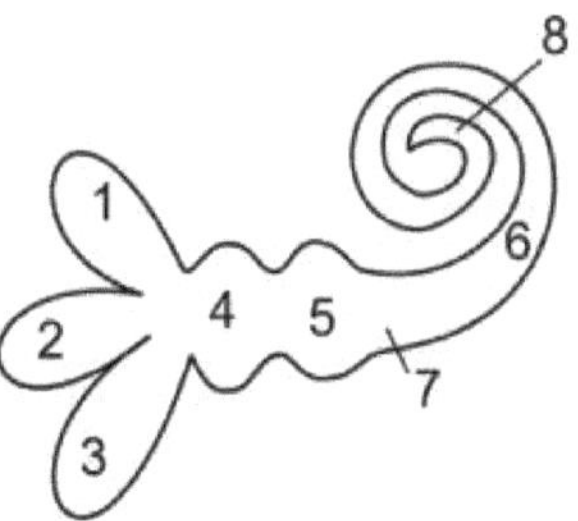

adequate stimulus is rectilinear accelerated and decelerated movements, jumping, shaking and head tilt.

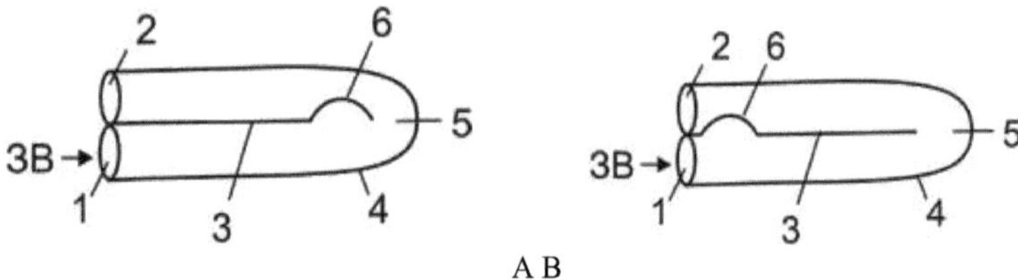

This diagram illustrates the mechanism of auditory sensation during the action of low (A) and high (B) frequency sound. During the action of low frequency sound (A) the whole perilymph column from the base of the cochlea (1) to its apex oscillates, so the bending of the main membrane (3) occurs in the region of the apex (5), which contributes to the excitation of neurons of Geschle's gyrus, leading to auditory sensations characteristic for the perception of low frequency sounds.

During the action of high frequency sound (B), perilymph oscillation occurs at the base of the cochlea, so the bending of the main membrane (3) occurs in the area of the base (6), which contributes to the excitation of neurons of the Geschle gyrus, leading to auditory sensations characteristic of the perception of high frequency sounds.

HIGHER NERVOUS ACTIVITY

Conditioned and unconditional reflexes

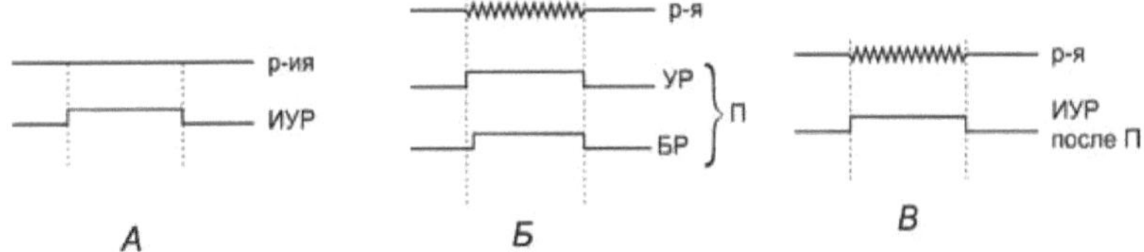

The diagram shows the method of development of a conditioned reflex - the organism's reaction to a conditioned (indifferent) stimulus with the obligatory participation of the cortex of the large hemispheres). When an isolated conditioned stimulus (ICS) is used, there is no reaction (A). In case of simultaneous action of the conditioned stimulus (SD) and unconditioned stimulus (CR) (P - reinforcement), there is a reaction (B). The appearance of a reaction at the action of an isolated conditioned stimulus (C) after repeated reinforcement (7-10 times) indicates the formation of a conditioned reflex.

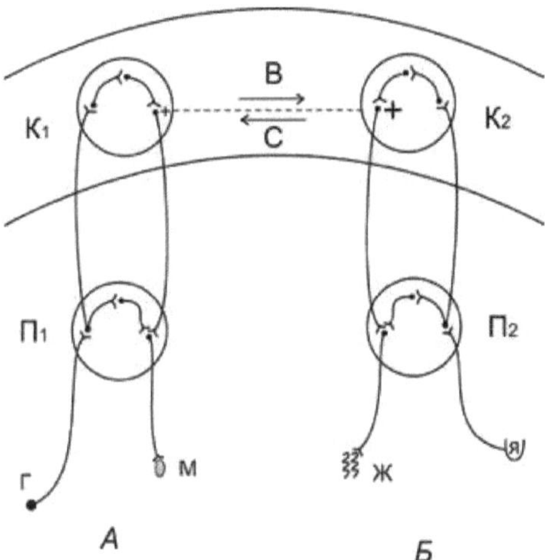

The diagram shows the mechanism of formation of a conditioned reflex. According to E. Asratyan's definition, a conditioned reflex is a synthesis of two or more unconditional reflexes. From this definition follows: 1) a conditioned reflex is carried out with the obligatory participation of the cortex of the large hemispheres - the PMA (synthesis is carried out in the PMA); 2) any conditioned reflex is carried out on the basis of an unconditioned reflex, so any unconditioned reflex can be conditioned. This scheme shows that two conditioned reflexes (A - blinking reflex, B - salivary release reflex) can be developed on the basis of two unconditional reflexes (blinking and salivary release reflexes). The blinking unconditioned reflex is realised by the action of a strong light stimulus. Blinking conditioned reflex is carried out on a weak food stimulus. Unconditional salivary reflex is carried out to a strong food stimulus, and the conditional salivary reflex - to a weak light stimulus. Let's consider the mechanism of occurrence of the conditioned salivary reflex. For this purpose, we carry out reinforcement in the following way: after a weak light stimulus (A) we act with a strong food stimulus (B). In this case, two foci of excitation (K1 - weak excitation and K2 - strong excitation) appear simultaneously in the PMA. According to the dominant principle, the weak excitation spreads towards the strong excitation (C). With repeated reinforcement in the cortex of the large hemispheres, a temporary connection between the two centres is formed. The formation of a temporary connection is evidenced by the presence of salivation on the isolated action of a weak light conditioned stimulus. In this case, the light stimulus causes excitation in the PMA (in the centre perceiving the conditioned stimulus - K1), which spreads through a temporary connection to the centre perceiving the food stimulus (K2), from here impulses arrive to the salivary glands and salivary reflex occurs.

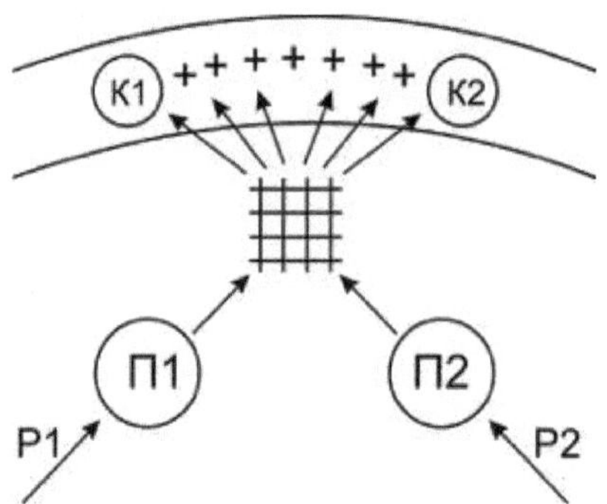

The diagram shows the mechanism of conditioned reflex emergence according to the convergent theory of P.K. Anokhin. The simultaneous action of conditioned (P1) and unconditioned (P2) stimuli (reinforcement) excites subcortical centres (P1 and P2) and as a result the reticular formation (RF) is involved in the process. From the RF there are two streams of impulses (convergence occurs) to the cortex of the large hemispheres, where excitation occurs simultaneously all the way from the centre perceiving the conditioned stimulus (K1) to the centre perceiving the unconditioned stimulus (K2). With repeated reinforcement, a temporal connection between K1 and K2 occurs in the large hemispheric cortex, resulting in a response to an isolated conditioned stimulus.

GND inhibition

The diagram reflects the types of inhibition in the cortex of the large hemispheres (1), i.e. higher nervous activity (HNA): 1) unconditional, or external inhibition (T1) is noted in neurons of the cortex of the large hemispheres (2,3); 2) conditional, or internal inhibition (T2), in which the

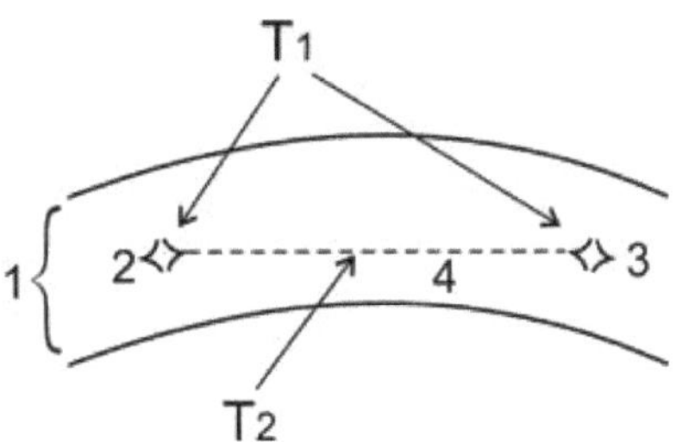

temporal connection disappears or is weakened (4). Unconditional inhibition includes: 1) external inhibition (permanent and extinguishing); 2) inhibitory, or guarding inhibition. Internal inhibition occurs as a result of the cessation of reinforcement after the development of a conditioned reflex. Depending on the method of cessation of reinforcement, the following types of internal inhibition are distinguished: 1) extinction inhibition; 2) differentiation inhibition; 3) delayed inhibition; 4) conditioned inhibition.

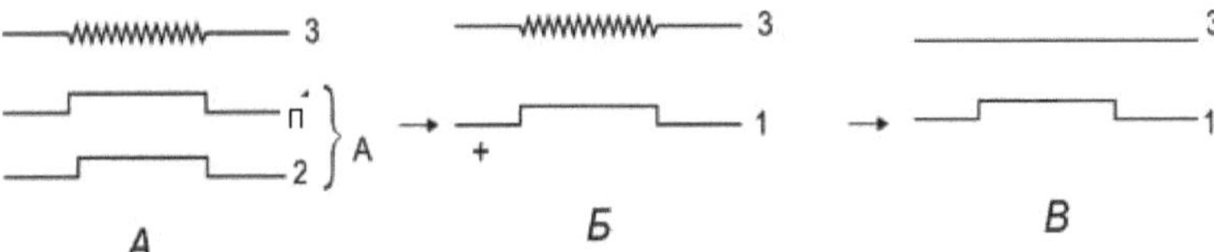

This figure shows the way in which the extinction of internal inhibition occurs. With repeated reinforcement (P) we produce a conditioned reflex (A). The occurrence of a conditioned reflex (B) is evidenced by the presence of a reaction (3) to the isiolated application of the conditioned stimulus (B-1). After the development of the conditioned reflex, we stop reinforcement completely and soon the catching reflex disappears (C), i.e. there is no reaction (B-3) to the isolated action of the conditioned stimulus (B-1).

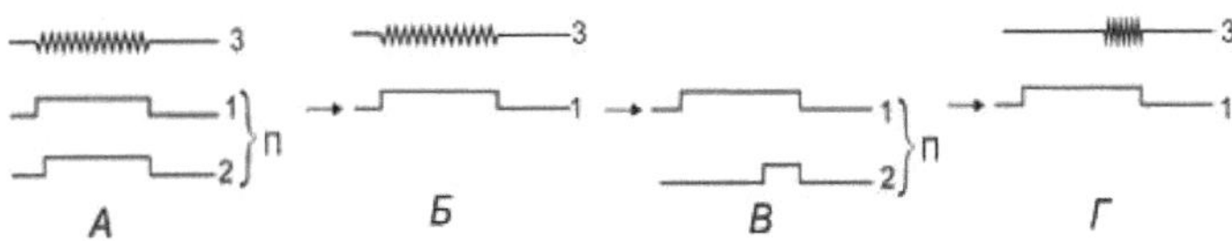

This figure shows the way in which delayed internal inhibition occurs. At repeated reinforcement (P) we produce a conditioned reflex (A). The occurrence of a conditioned reflex (B) is evidenced by the presence of a reaction to the isiolated application of the conditioned stimulus (B-1). After the development of the conditioned reflex, we continue to periodically reinforce the action of the conditioned stimulus with the action of the unconditioned stimulus, but with a long delay (C). After periodic delayed reinforcement, isolated action of the conditioned stimulus causes a delayed response (D).

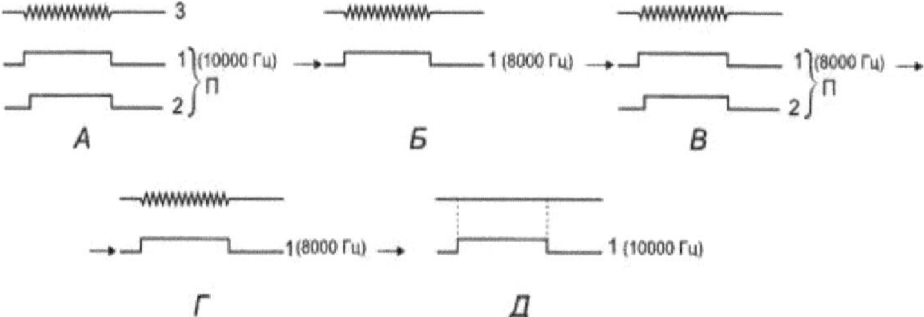

This figure shows the way of occurrence of differentiation internal inhibition. With repeated reinforcement (P) we develop a conditioned reflex to the sound 10000 Hz (A). After the development of the conditioned reflex, the reaction occurs to the action of the sound of 8000 Hz (B). In the future, the action of the 10000 Hz sound will be periodically reinforced by the action of the unconditioned stimulus (C), and the action of the 8000 Hz sound will not be reinforced. As a result, the reaction only to 10000 Hz is preserved (D), and the reaction to the sound of 8000 Hz disappears (E), i.e. differentiation inhibition occurs.

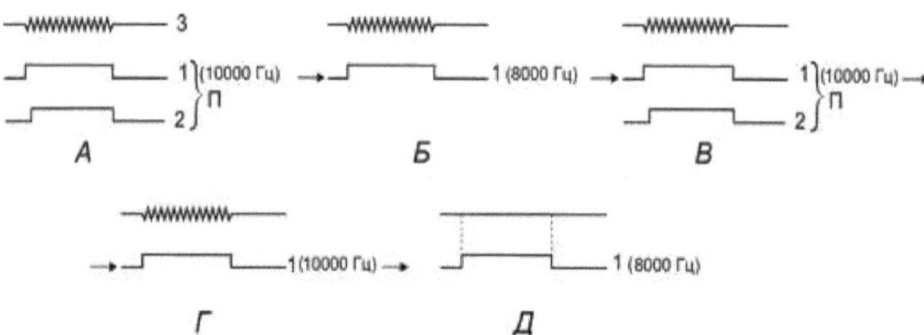

This figure shows the way of occurrence of conditioned internal inhibition. With repeated reinforcement (P) we develop a conditioned reflex to a light stimulus (A). After development of the conditioned reflex, the reaction occurs at simultaneous action of light and sound conditioned stimuli (B). In the future, the action of the light stimulus will be periodically reinforced by the action of the unconditional stimulus (C), and in case of simultaneous action of light and sound we will not reinforce it. As a result, the reaction only to the action of the conditioned light stimulus is preserved (D), and to the simultaneous action of light and sound the reaction disappears (E), i.e. there is a conditioned internal inhibition.

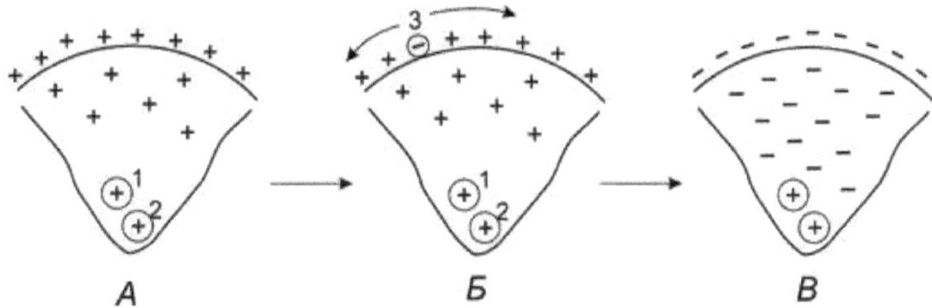

This diagram shows the mechanism of sleep according to I.P. Pavlov. In the awake state, the cerebral cortex and subcortical structures of the brain are in an active state (A). Under the action of a prolonged auditory or visual stimulus, local inhibition (B-3) occurs in the HPA, which irradiates throughout the cortex. As a result of irradiation, inhibition covers the entire PMA and subcortical structures with the exception of vital centres (1,2) - respiratory and vasomotor - sleep occurs. Thus, according to I.P. Pavlov, sleep is a spilt inhibition of the HPA and subcortical structures of the brain with preservation of excitation of vital centres.

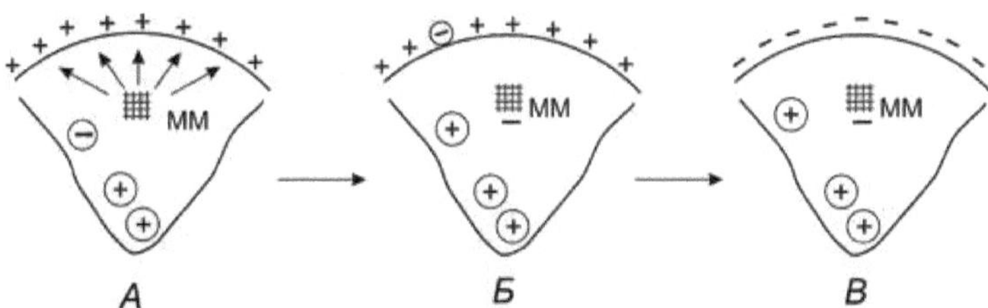

This diagram shows the mechanism of sleep according to P.K. Anokhin. In the awake state, the cerebral cortex and subcortical structures of the brain are in an active state (A) due to excitation of the Magoon-Moruci centre of the brain reticular formation (MM). At the same time, the Hess centre in the hypothalamus (D) is in a state of inhibition. Under the action of a prolonged auditory or visual stimulus, local inhibition (B-3) occurs in the PMA, due to which the Hess centre is excited and the MM centre is inhibited. As a result, the flow of active impulses from the MM centre to the PMA stops, and there is a spilt inhibition of the PMA and subcortical structures of the brain with the exception of vital centres (1,2 - respiratory and vasomotor) and the Hess centre - sleep occurs.

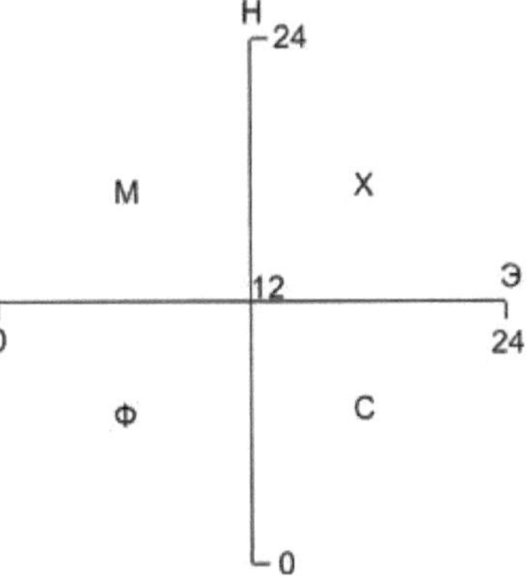

Types of GND

This scheme reflects the method of determining extraversion-introversion according to Eysenck, types of GND according to I.P. Pavlov and temperaments according to Hypo-Krat. The abscissa axis reflects the degree of extraversion expression: the number of points from 0 to 11 - these are introverts; from 13 to 24 - these are extroverts. The ordinate axis reflects the degree of neuro-ticism (stability of nervous processes in the cortex of the large hemispheres): the number of points from 0 to 11 - with stable nervous processes; from 13 to 24 - with unstable nervous processes. The Eysenck scale of extraversion-introversion reflects the property of mobility of nervous processes according to I.P. Pavlov. The Eysenck scale of neuroticism reflects the property of balance of nervous processes according to I.P. Pavlov. The right lower square testifies to a stable extrovert (sanguine according to Hippocrates, strong mobile, balanced type according to I.P.Pavlov). The right upper square testifies to an unstable extravert (choleric according to Hippocrates, strong mobile, unbalanced type according to I.P.Pavlov). The left bottom square testifies about stable introvert (phlegmatic according to Hippocrates, strong sedentary, balanced type according to I.P.Pavlov). The left upper square indicates an unstable introvert (melancholic according to Hippocrates, weak type according to I.P.Pavlov).

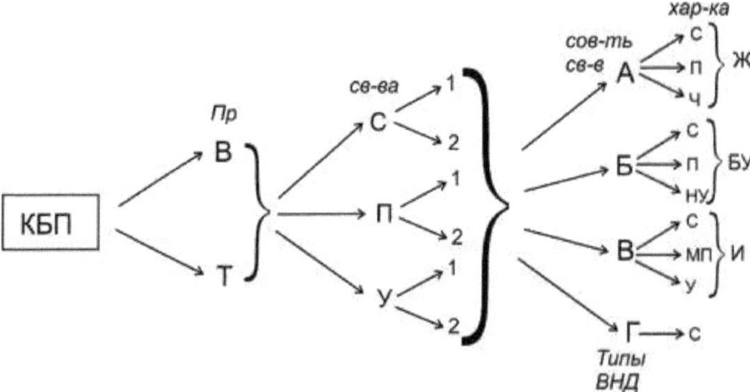

This diagram shows a brief characterisation of the types of the AND according to I.P. Pavlov. In the cortex of the large hemispheres (LHB) there are two processes (P) - excitation (E) and inhibition (T). Each of these processes is characterised by three properties (sv-va): strength (C), mobility (P - speed of change of excitation process by inhibition and vice versa), equilibrium (U - determined by the correspondence of the strength of excitatory and inhibitory processes). By each property separately all people are divided into two types (1,2): by strength - strong and weak; by mobility - mobile and sedentary (inert); by equilibrium - balanced and unbalanced (unrestrained). According to the totality of the three properties (the combination of properties) all people can be divided into four types of GND (A, B, C, D). Characteristic (characteristic) of type A - strong (c), mobile (p) and balanced (y), or lively (L). Type B - strong (c), mobile (p) and unbalanced (nu), or unrestrained (BU). Type C - strong (c),little mobile (mp) and balanced (u), or inert(I). Type D - weak (s).

This table shows the interaction of types of GND according to Pavlov, extraversion-introversion according to Eysenck and temperaments according to Hippocrates. Hippocrates distinguished four temperaments by the ratio of different body fluids: sanguine (Sa), choleric (X), phlegmatic (F) and melancholic (M). I.P. Pavlov distinguished four types of GND by the properties of excitation and inhibition processes in the PMA. I.P. Pavlov distinguished three properties: strength of excitatory and inhibitory processes (S), mobility (M) and equilibrium of these processes (E). As can be seen from the table, the first type (I) is strong, mobile and balanced, or calm; the second type (II) is strong, mobile, but unbalanced with the predominance of excitation processes, or unrestrained; the third type (III) is strong sedentary and balanced, or inert; the fourth type (IV) is weak, that is, all properties are weakly expressed. Eysenck has allocated two properties for characterisation of types of people: 1) expression of extraversion-introversion (E) on which all people can be divided into extraverts and introverts; 2) neuroticism (N), i.e. stability of nervous processes on which all people can be divided into stable and unstable. According to the totality of these properties all people can be divided into four types: 1) stable extrovert; 2) unstable extrovert; 3) stable introvert; 4) unstable introvert. The table shows that extroversion- introversion according to Eysenck corresponds to the mobility of nervous processes according to I.P. Pavlov, and neuroticism according to Eysenck corresponds to the equilibrium of nervous processes according to I.P. Pavlov. Thus, the first type according to I.P. Pavlov is a sanguine according to Hippocrates, or a stable extrovert according to Eysenck; the second type according to I.P. Pavlov is a choleric according to Hippocrates, or an unstable extrovert according to Eysenck; the third type according to I.P. Pavlov is a sanguine according to I.P. Pavlov.The third type according to I.P. Pavlov is phlegmatic according to Hippocrates, or stable introvert according to Eysenck; the fourth type according to I.P. Pavlov is melancholic according to Hippocrates, or unstable introvert according to Eysenck.

Типы / Св-ва			I	II	III	IV
П А В Л О В	С		+	+	+	−
	П		+	+	−	−
	У		+	−	+	−
АЙЗЕНК	Э	Э	+	+	−	−
		И	−	−	+	+
	Н	С	+	−	+	+
		НС	−	+	−	+
ГИПОКРАТ			С	Х	Ф	М

EMOTIONS, BIOLOGICAL MOTIVATIONS AND STRESS

The physiology of emotion

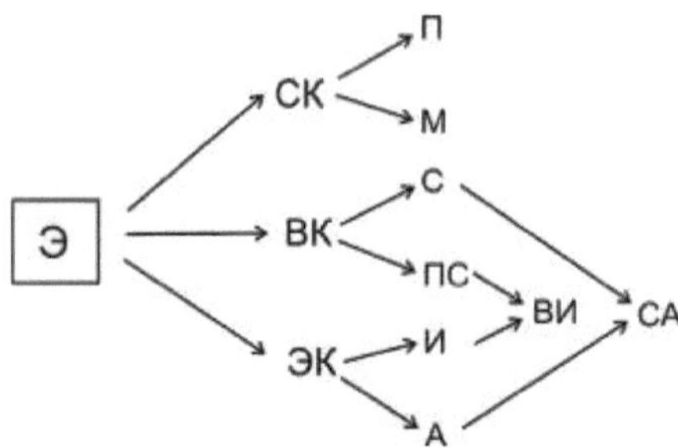

A scheme reflecting the components of emotion (E). Any emotion includes the following components: 1) somatic component (SC) due to changes in the tone of muscles of the trunk and limbs (in this case the posture of a person in space changes - P), as well as changes in the tone of mimic muscles (in this case the facial expression of a person changes (M); 2) vegetative component (VC) due to changes in the tone of sympathetic (S) and parsympathetic (PS) sections of the autonomous nervous system (ANS); 3) endocrine component (EC) due to changes in the function of the pancreas (change in the concentration of insulin in the blood - I) and the brain layer of the adrenal glands (change in the concentration of adrenaline and noradrenaline in the blood - A). Activation of the sympathetic section of the ANS is usually accompanied by activation of the function of the brain layer of the adrenal glands, i.e. activation of the sympathoadrenal system (SA). Activation of the parasympathetic ANS is accompanied by activation of the pancreas, i.e. activation of the vago-insulin system (VI).

Biological motivations

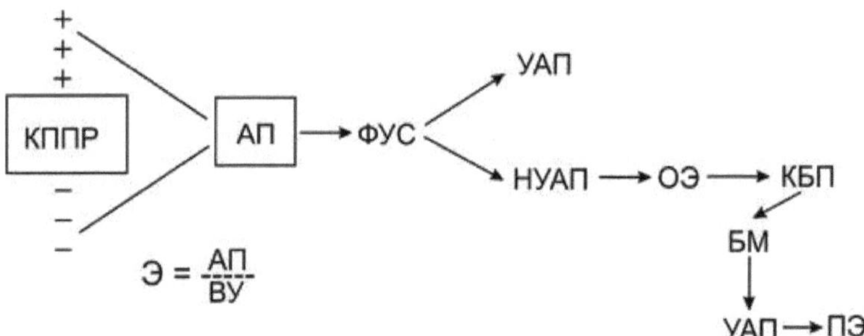

$$Э = \frac{АП}{ВУ}$$

The diagram shows the formation of negative (NE) and positive (PE) emotions from the perspective of functional systems of the organism. At first, there is a deviation of any final useful adaptive result (KPPP) from the optimal level in the direction of decrease or in the direction bof increase - this leads to the formation of the actual need of the organism (NA), the satisfaction of which (UAP) can be realised at the expense of the internal reserve of the corresponding functional system (FUS). If at inclusion of all effectors of the FUS there is no satisfaction of the actual internal need (NIAP), a negative emotion arises (a signal about the necessity to include in the work of the FUS an external link - behaviour), excitation from the hypothalamus passes to the cortex of the large hemispheres due to what biological motivation occurs (BM - a purposeful behavioural act). If BM satisfies an actual need of the organism, a positive emotion (PE) occurs, if BM does not satisfy AP, the negative emotion persists. From the point of view of functional systems of an organism emotion (E) is a relation of actual need (AP) to probability of satisfaction (PI) of this need (E=AP/PI). Thus, the biological role of negative emotions is that their occurrence testifies to impossibility of satisfaction of AP by functional reserves of an organism and necessity of performance of purposeful behaviour. In this case, one behaviour is replaced by another until the actual need is satisfied. An indicator of AP satisfaction is the appearance of a positive emotion.

Mechanism of stress

$$С → К → Г → КЛБ → ПдГ → АКТГ → КНП → КСТ → ТК → ПУ$$

This scheme reflects the sequence of processes occurring under stress (C), a humoral mechanism that increases tissue resistance (TR). Stress (C) affects the cerebral cortex (C), from where impulses flow to the hypothalamus (H). The hypothalamus secretes corticoliberin (CLB), which affects the anterior lobe of the pituitary gland (PdH). The anterior lobe of the pituitary gland secretes adrenocorticotropic hormone (ACTH), which humourally influences the adrenal cortex (ACP). The adrenal cortex secretes corticosteroids (ACTH), which humorally influence body tissues (TC) resulting in increased resistance to stress (STS).

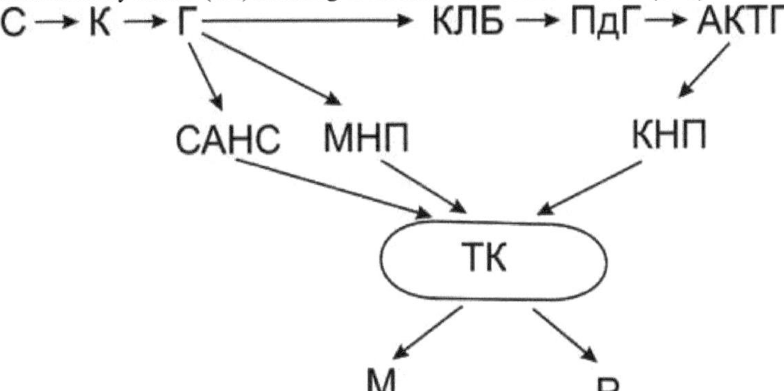

The diagram shows the nervous and humoral mechanism of mobilisation (M) and resistance (R) of functional systems of the organism (FUS) under stress. Stress (C) acts on the cortex of the large hemispheres (K), from where impulses go to the hypothalamus. As a result, there is a nervous and humoral influence of the hypothalamus on the FUS. The hypothalamus secretes corticoliberin (CLB), which influences the anterior lobe of the pituitary gland (PdH). The anterior lobe of the pituitary gland secretes adrenocorticotropic hormone (ACTH), which humourally influences the adrenal cortex (ACP). The adrenal cortex secretes corticosteroids, which humorally affect the tissues of the body (TC) as a result of increasing their resistance (resistance) to the action of stress (P). At the same time through efferent pathways nerve impulses reach the adrenal medulla (AMP), dopamine, norepinephrine and adrenaline (catecholamines) are released, acting on tissues as a result of mobilisation of FUS (M). In addition, the hypothalamus increases the tone of the sympathetic section of the autonomic nervous system (SANS), which also leads to the mobilisation of FUS. Thus, under the action of stress there is mobilisation of FUS due to the activation of the sympathoadrenal system (increase in the tone of the SANS and enhancement of the function of the brain layer of the adrenal glands) and increase in the resistance (stability) of these systems.

Stress-realising systems

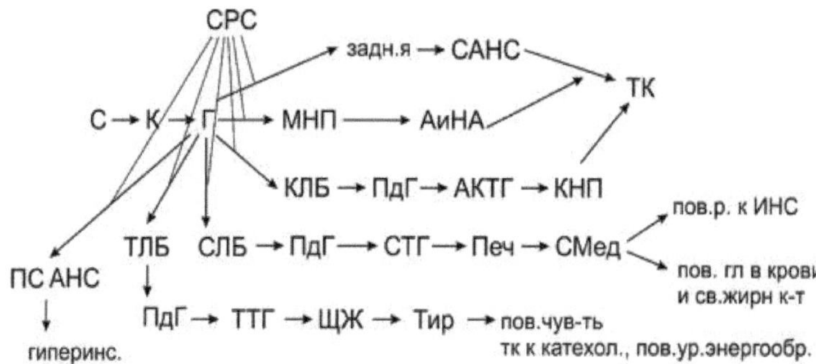

This diagram shows the mechanism of activation of the stress-releasing system (SRS) under the action of stress (C) on the organism. Stress (C) influences the cortex of the large hemispheres (K) and through it the hypothalamus, which leads to the activation of the SRS: 1) there is excitation of the posterior nuclei of the hypothalamus, i.e. activation of the sympathetic section of the autonomic nervous system (SANS), which is accompanied by mobilisation of the cardiovascular system, respiration and skeletal muscles; 2) nerve action on the medullary layer of the adrenal gland (MLA), which leads to the release of adrenaline and noradrenaline into the blood, resulting in an increase in BP, cardiac output, free fatty acids and glucose levels. These two systems (1,2) are often combined as the sympathoadrenal system; 3) activation of the adrenocortical system: release of corticoliberin (CLB) affecting the anterior lobe of the pituitary gland. The release of adrenocorticotropic hormone (ACTH) increases, which through the adrenal cortex increases the release of glucocorticoids. These hormones significantly increase the body's energy reserves - glucose and free fatty acid levels increase. In addition, ACTH increases the production of aldosterone, which initially increases the reabsorption of sodium ions and through the pivotally countercurrent system increases the reabsorption of water, which ultimately increases

BP; 4) activation of the somatotropic system: the release of somatoliberin (SLB), affecting the anterior lobe of the pituitary gland (PdH). The release of somatotropic hormone (STH) increases, which through the liver (Pech) increases the release of somatomedins (Smed), which leads to increased resistance to insulin, accelerated mobilisation of stored fats in the body - increases the content of glucose in the blood and free fatty acids; 5) activation of the thyroid system: release of thyrolyberin (TLB), affecting the anterior lobe of the pituitary gland (PdH). Thyrotropic hormone (TTH) release increases, which through the thyroid gland (thyroid) increases the release of thyroxine and triiodothyrosine (Tir), which leads to increased sensitivity to catecholamines, the level of energy formation increases; 6) the activity of the parasympathetic system of the autonomic nervous system (PSANS) increases, which leads to hyperinsulinaemia.

TABLE OF CONTENTS

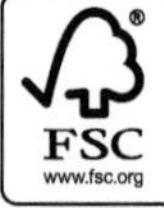

Printed by Books on Demand GmbH, Norderstedt / Germany